Praise

The Ultimate Guide to Prostate Pleasure

"This modern guide will steer you past any hang-ups and gently around anatomy's curves to bring you prostate pleasure and orgasmic thrills you never knew you had coming to you. If you've got questions, Charlie and Aislinn have got the answers."

—Dr. Sadie Allison, author of
Tickle My Tush: Mild-To-Wild Analplay Adventures for Everybooty

"A great addition to a largely underground history that is finally coming into the light. Everyone deserves the sex information that will make their desires consensually possible, safe, and full of pleasure."

—Dr. Carol Queen, staff sexologist at
Good Vibrations and author of *Real Live Nude Girl*

"This superb guide combines the friendliness of a good buddy with the savvy knowledge of a top-notch sex educator, explaining the ins and outs, hows and whys, of prostate pleasure, including answering those questions you thought you couldn't ask anybody. Whatever you want to know about the pleasures and the how-tos of prostate stimulation, it's in this book."

—Joan Price, author of
Naked at Our Age: Talking Out Loud About Senior Sex

"Dr. Charlie Glickman and Aislinn Emirzian have written the end-all guide to prostate pleasure. This book will appeal to so many different groups of people—solo, partnered, vanilla, hetero, queer, bi, gay, young, old—everyone who wants to know more about this oft-ignored source of pleasure in one's sexual repertoire. The focus of this book is on informing beginners through the master level, with everything from dispelling myths to basic communication skills to the how-tos of giving or receiving prostate pleasure. Well done!"

—Lanae St.John,
sexologist and sex educator at TheMamaSutra.net

The Ultimate Guide to Prostate Pleasure

The Ultimate Guide to Prostate Pleasure

Erotic Exploration for Men and Their Partners

**CHARLIE GLICKMAN, PhD
and AISLINN EMIRZIAN**

**Foreword by
CAROL QUEEN, PhD**

**Afterword by
DEBBY HERBENICK, PhD, MPH**

CLEiS
PRESS

Published in the United States by Cleis Press, Inc.,
2246 Sixth St., Berkeley, California 94710.

Printed in the United States.
Cover design: Scott Idleman/Blink
Cover photograph: Loungepark
Text design: Frank Wiedemann

First Edition.
10 9 8 7 6 5 4 3 2 1

Trade paper ISBN: 978-1-57344-904-5
E-book ISBN: 978-1-57344-921-2

Library of Congress Cataloging-in-Publication Data

Glickman, Charlie.
 The ultimate guide to prostate pleasure : erotic exploration for men and their partners /
Charlie Glickman and Aislinn Emirzian. -- 1st ed.
     p. cm.
 Includes bibliographical references and index.
 ISBN 978-1-57344-904-5 (pbk. : alk. paper)
 1. Sex instruction. 2. Prostate. 3. Anal sex. 4. Sexual excitement. I. Emirzian, Aislinn. II.
Title.

 HQ31.G656 2013
 613.9071--dc23

                              2012040224

TABLE OF CONTENTS

ILLUSTRATIONS

FOREWORD

Even though we live in a time when anal sex movies are available at just a mouse click, anal pleasure—especially for men—remains a topic about which most people have never received good information. Sex education as a whole, in fact, doesn't serve to promote or explore pleasure; people have to figure that part out on their own, and many don't have time, ready access to information, or even the understanding that sex could feel better to them than it does right now. Still others cannot, for personal reasons, prioritize pleasure—after all, we are still getting mainstream messages that sex is primarily for reproduction, though that is hardly the only sexual message we hear. It has become a very lively discussion, if you know where to look for alternative perspectives.

Still, male anal pleasure and prostate play lie far outside the charmed circle of what many people understand sex to be, and anyone seeking to explore it needs to find a source of knowledge. This information mostly used to be in the hands of men who had sex with men: open discussion of anal sex and prostate play was far easier to find in the gay community, despite the irony that (as one study noted) more married heterosexual women, percentage-wise, engaged in anal intercourse than gay men. Jack Morin, in his book *Anal Pleasure and Health*, brought this information to anyone who needed it—but still, when my partner Dr. Robert Morgan Lawrence and I began traveling and teaching anal play workshops at the dawn of the 1990s, most people did not even know there was an informational infrastructure to be had. It has been a huge privilege for Robert and me to talk and teach about anal pleasure, for no knowledge is as welcome as knowledge that once seemed unobtainable.

With Robert, who had been teaching anal eroticism skills since the 1970s, I appeared in *Bend Over Boyfriend*—essentially a video distillation of his knowledge—which helped innumerable curious couples explore back-door delights. This became one of the best selling movies Good Vibrations ever carried. If it was not clear before that there existed plenty of pent-up desire for male anal play (and information about anal pleasure in general), this response, and feedback from many, many men and their partners, has definitely shown otherwise.

The fact is, all kinds of men love prostate stimulation and pleasure; even when they do not share this predilection with their partners, they may engage in solo anal play. Other men have decided to explore it in the hope that prostate massage will help keep them healthy. And increasingly, people with prostates are sharing erotic explorations with their partners. This book supports all of them—as well as the curious who haven't yet put their ass on the line for erotic enjoyment—with permission, knowledge, safety information, and suggested play styles. It's a great addition to a largely underground history that is finally coming into the light. Everyone deserves the sex information that will make their desires consensually possible, safe, and full of pleasure.

Carol Queen, PhD
San Francisco

INTRODUCTION

The prostate has been getting a lot of attention lately. Coyote Days, toy buyer for Good Vibrations, says, "In the years that I've been buyer, there's definitely been more emphasis, focus, and attention directed toward prostate stimulation." According to Christine Fawley of PleasureMechanics.com, "Prostate massage is the hottest trend in male sexuality, as straight men all around the world are waking up to the potential pleasures of anal play and prostate stimulation." What's all the buzz about?

Curiosity about the health benefits of prostate massage has inspired lots of men to try it out and to discover some pleasant side effects—intense pleasure and orgasm. Many others have been intrigued to hear that it is possible to have an orgasm through prostate massage that feels completely different from what they are used to from penile stimulation, and that this can happen without touching their cock at all. Not to mention multiple orgasms and full-body orgasms that some men experience through prostate play!

In recent years, people have been calling the prostate the "male G-spot," a term that is suggestive of how powerful this hidden pleasure zone can be. And while the prostate has been common knowledge for a long time among gay men and other sexual subcultures, the increased mainstream popularity of pegging (strap-on sex for male–female couples, with the male as the receiver) has led many hetero couples to discover the intense sensations that this area can offer.

As the reputation of the prostate has grown, so has the curiosity of men and their partners. More and more ears are perking up to the whispers and shouts about prostate massage as a source of intense erotic sensation. In our work as sexuality educators, we've fielded more questions from men and their partners about prostate stimulation than we can keep track of.

With the increasing buzz about the prostate, more sex guides ranging from Tantra books to sex toy guides mention the prostate as an erogenous zone. However, most only mention it in passing, and don't elaborate much further than to say "Insert fingers and curl them toward the front of the body." Given the significant popular demand for information and the very limited number of comprehensive guides to prostate stimulation, we decided to write a detailed guide to finding and enjoying the prostate by yourself or with a partner.

Since you're reading this, odds are that you're curious about prostate play. Maybe you've been thinking of trying it out. Maybe you've given it a shot and want some new tips. Or perhaps your partner is interested and you're willing to learn more. However you got here, we're glad you did. Unlike some other sexual practices, trying prostate play often presents hurdles. Concerns about anal play, safety, cleanliness, sexual orientation, masculinity, and gender roles can hold men and their partners back. Or simply never having heard much about the prostate as a pleasure zone can keep lots of people from exploring it. We're always excited to help people discover new ways to experience pleasure, so we give you all the information you need to know to relax and enjoy yourself.

All Genders and Orientations Are Doing This

All kinds of people get into prostate play. We have personally spoken with men of all different orientations—straight, gay, bi, queer, pansexual, etc.—who get into prostate play by themselves, with a partner, or both. It is a very diverse group of people that enjoys prostate play!

Despite the rather tenacious idea that anal penetration isn't something heterosexual men do (as receivers), we've talked with enough hetero men and female partners to know that's simply not true. But because male-receptive anal penetration is still very taboo outside gay male circles and sex-positive subcultures, the enjoyment of prostate play (and male-receptive anal play generally) by hetero men is not discussed as openly, and there is less awareness of these practices in the larger culture.

Even as more and more straight men and their partners are trying this out, many straight men and their partners still would be surprised by the suggestion that he could enjoy having his prostate massaged during anal penetration, and that she could enjoy doing it. Quite a few people only know of the prostate in connection with cancer, and lots of guys are uncomfortable with the idea of anal penetration anyway. One of our main goals with this book was to reach as many straight men as possible and give them all the info they need to enjoy prostate play.

We also tried to make the book relevant to men who sleep with men. Many men who are part of a strong gay/bi/queer/pansexual community are already fairly knowledgeable about the prostate; this information is typically passed around between partners and in the community at large, since anal penetration is frequently normalized in these circles. Still, we hope that our readers who are gay/bi/queer/pansexual men might learn something new.

In addition to the pleasures of receiving prostate stimulation, people of all genders who are partners to men can enjoy being on the giving end of prostate play with fingers, toys, or a cock or strap-on dildo. Throughout the book, we dance back and forth between addressing those who are looking for their own prostate and those who would like to learn to pleasure someone else's. Also, we gave special attention to women who want to pleasure a man's prostate, as we think this information is in high demand among many women who play with men.

Lastly, though this book is addressed to men and their

partners, it's important to note that transgender women have a prostate too. (Actually, everyone has a prostate—see chapter 3, What Is the Prostate?) Plenty of transgender women enjoy having their prostate stimulated. Others find that they don't enjoy it for a variety of reasons. For those who do find it pleasurable, the techniques are mostly the same as those for cisgender men (men whose experience of gender is aligned with the gender they were assigned at birth). There are also some important differences; we describe these in the sidebar "Prostate Pleasure for Transgender Women" in chapter 2, The Sexy Prostate.

What You'll Find Inside

We begin by addressing common concerns with a chapter on FAQs, where we briefly list and respond to the most common questions and concerns we have encountered in talking with men about prostate play. Next, we explain the role of the prostate in male reproductive anatomy and discuss the erogenous nature of the prostate.

After that, we get into the how-to section of the book: anal play and hygiene, the basics of pleasurable anal penetration, how to find the prostate, and what to do once you have. In addition to an in-depth description of solo and partnered massage technique, we cover toys and anal intercourse/strap-on sex. In the final portion of the book, we focus on some of the larger issues that can affect prostate play: how ideas of masculinity can hold men back; prostate health; and some of the ways in which prostate massage is believed to benefit health.

Even if you think you know everything you need to know

about a particular topic, we invite you to take a look at the relevant chapter. We thought we knew a lot before we started writing this book—we were surprised to discover how much more there was to know. You might be too!

And just as with anything about sex, nothing we describe here works for everyone. We invite you to try out as many different approaches as you want, but don't get discouraged if some of them aren't your thing. We have plenty of other suggestions.

A Note about Language

One of the hardest tasks in writing about sex is deciding what terms to use for body parts. Some people prefer terms like *penis* and *anus*, while others find them too medical or clinical. On the other hand, words like *cock* or *asshole*, more comfortable for some, are too slangy or offensive to others. There's no way to talk about sex that's guaranteed to suit everyone all the time.

We decided to use different terms in different places. For example, when we're talking about medical issues related to the prostate, we shift into more medical language. In other places, we keep it more informal. But there's nothing better about one term or another. It's just a matter of preference.

Here is one term we'll define right away: *P-spot*. The prostate, as we explain in chapter 3, What Is the Prostate?, is an erogenous zone very similar to the erogenous zone in women known as the "G-spot." Some sexuality educators and prostate play enthusiasts have started calling the prostate "the P-spot," both to highlight that similarity and because they think it's a sexier word than *prostate*. We use both terms in different places, and you're welcome to use whichever you're more comfortable with. In fact, we encourage you to come up with new names for this erogenous zone, if any should strike your fancy!

Who We Are and How This Book Came Together

Charlie has been a sexuality educator for over 20 years in a variety of settings; in 2005 he received his PhD in Adult Sexuality Education from the Union Institute and University. He has created workshops on many different sexual practices and communities. He teaches courses on sexuality for local universities, presents at conferences and other events, and writes a lot about sexual topics. He'd been teaching workshops and talking with people about prostate play for a while before writing this book. He has worked at Good Vibrations since 1996, starting out in the stores and eventually becoming the Education Program Manager.

We met when Aislinn was hired at Good Vibrations as a Sex Educator–Sales Associate. Aislinn began sex ed as a college student, where she was part of a peer sex ed group that taught workshops to fellow students. After graduation, she got involved with sex-positive adult toy stores, beginning with Oh My Sensuality Shop in Massachusetts, and later moving to San Francisco to work for Good Vibrations. During her years as a sex educator, she has taught workshops on subjects including the G-spot, queer pornography, sex parties for women, and, of course, the prostate.

Between us, we've talked with hundreds of men and their

partners about prostate play. In addition to these informal conversations, we conducted two online surveys to find out more. The first focused on technique. Seventy-five people responded—givers and receivers, of all sexual orientations and levels of experience—saying what they like and don't like, how they include prostate play in their sexual relationships, and sharing lots of useful tips. The second survey focused on sensation, and it was just for the receivers. This gave us great insight into how men experience this pleasure, what it actually feels like for them. The generosity of all these respondents in sharing the details of their sex lives with us was tremendously useful and we're deeply grateful to everyone who participated. This book wouldn't have been complete without you!

A Big Thanks

Writing this book has been an amazing experience, and we couldn't have done it without lots of help. Our partners, Michael and Elizabeth, listened to us geek out about the prostate for months. Thanks for your support. Also, a special thanks to our friends Margaret Brown and Stephanie Edd for their assistance in locating scholarly articles.

We're also deeply grateful for all the experts, medical professionals, and colleagues who answered our questions, checked our information, kept us up to date on recent research, and offered feedback. A big thank-you to Alan Shindel, Carol Queen, Robert Lawrence, Myrtle Wilhite, Beverly Whipple, Jonathan Branfman, Susan Stiritz, Jan Robinson, Stephanie Prendergast, Leah Alchin, The Source School of Tantra, and Charles Muir.

BEFORE WE START: FREQUENTLY ASKED QUESTIONS

So you've decided to give prostate play a try. Or maybe you've done it before and you want to learn some new tricks. We think that's great! More men and their partners are discovering how much pleasure this often-overlooked part of the body can bring them.

Before we get into the how-to side of things, there are some matters we want to address first. Many men have questions and concerns about prostate play, and these questions can hold them back. Here we address some of the most common concerns and FAQs of prostate enthusiasts. Maybe you've had some of these concerns in the past, or they're coming up for you now. We hope this chapter will help you feel more comfortable with exploring your prostate. And if you're a partner of a guy who wants to explore prostate play, you might find something useful here too.

"So my prostate gland is...up my ass?"

No, the prostate gland is not located in the rectum—it just happens to live next door! The prostate is a part of your reproductive anatomy. It's an "accessory sex gland" that contributes a portion of the fluid that makes up your semen. It surrounds the urethra, just behind and slightly above the bulb of the penis, a few inches inside the perineum (the area between your balls and your anus).

Like other parts of your sex equipment, the prostate can feel amazing when stimulated. However, because it is located inside the pelvis, it is less readily available for stimulation than your cock and balls.

Since the prostate happens to sit directly in front of the rectum, you can stimulate it by inserting a finger into the anus and stroking toward the front of the body. The rectal wall is thick enough to withstand gentle pressure, but thin enough that the pressure is easily transferred to the prostate on the other side.

The anal route is the most direct way to stimulate the prostate, so it's the preferred technique of many P-spot enthusiasts. But the prostate is not a part of your anal anatomy, and the ass is not the only available path. You can also massage the prostate indirectly by pressing upward through the perineum. Men have also reported feeling pleasurable prostate sensations during arousal, orgasm, and ejaculation, while flexing pelvic muscles, while fantasizing, and during a bowel movement.

"Isn't it messy?"

Uneasiness about making a mess was the number one concern mentioned by prostate enthusiasts we've heard from, regardless of sexual orientation. During anal penetration, it's certainly possible to come into contact with stuff that you might prefer not to. But most of the time, it's not so messy as you might imagine. And fortunately, it's pretty easy to minimize the mess factor.

Stool isn't stored in the rectum. It's stored deeper in the digestive tract, and only passes through the rectum on its way

"Just get over it! It feels awesome."

out. So between bowel movements, there usually isn't very much left behind. Sometimes stool remains in the rectum, especially if your diet is lacking in fiber, if you have loose stool, or if you use medications that affect your digestion. But most of the time there is little or no visible shit on toys or fingers after penetration, and little or no offensive odor in the air during play.

Still, if you are concerned, there are many ways to keep your play relatively clean and hygienic, such as wearing gloves, laying a towel on the bed, and rinsing out beforehand with an enema. (See chapter 4, Hygiene, for more information.)

Even with all these tips, there's always a chance that you'll come into contact with some feces. It's not the end of the world. As the bumper sticker says, "shit happens." Simply wipe it up and move on.

"Doesn't it hurt?"

Lots of people have had painful experiences with anal penetration. However, this usually happens because they were doing too much too soon: forcing entry, taking an object that was too big, or not using enough lube. Likewise, prostate massage can be painful if you press too hard or poke roughly in your eagerness to produce sensation. But most people can learn to receive anal penetration and prostate massage without pain.

If you are new at this, you might experience some discomfort and prostate tenderness during your first few forays. With a little practice, that usually goes away. But you can avoid pain entirely by following one simple rule: If it hurts, don't do it! This may mean taking your time and going more slowly and gently than you might prefer, but it's worth it to avoid the pain. (See chapter 5, Penetration 101, for tips on painless entry.)

"If a man gets penetrated, doesn't that mean he's gay/effeminate/being dominated?"

A lot of men are curious to find their prostate and see how it feels, but they hesitate because they are afraid that being penetrated would be in conflict with their masculinity. The story goes like this: "Only homos and sissies get fucked. Penetration is an act of domination. A real man doesn't get fucked—he does the fucking."

In short, we don't buy that. We have personally spoken to men from all over the masculinity spectrum and men of many different sexual orientations who love prostate play. You may not hear about it because (with the exception of some sexual subcultures) it's pretty hush-hush, but that doesn't mean it isn't happening!

The prostate is a part of your sex equipment and can be a source of great pleasure—whether you're doing this with a woman, with a man, or by yourself. That's why plenty of men of all orientations and all degrees of masculinity/femininity are into prostate play.

Not convinced? Check out chapter 13, Real Men Don't, and you'll find our explanation of where these negative ideas come from and why they are total nonsense. If these concerns are getting in your way, now might be a good time to skip ahead to that chapter before you read any further.

"Won't people think I'm weird?"

Some might—so don't tell them! Lots of others think it's A-OK. Just because some people may be uncomfortable with the idea of prostate play doesn't mean that there's anything wrong with it.

The sexual practices that are considered "weird" or "perverted" are always evolving. In the 50s, oral sex was a scandalous affair—think how commonplace (even vanilla!) that practice is considered today. Anal sex with a woman receiving was also quite taboo in recent decades, but now it's very common for women to try it and enjoy it. Who knows? Maybe in 10 or 20 years, male receptive anal penetration and prostate massage will be passé and some other kind of play will be the new taboo.

The point is, whether or not the kind of sex you have is "weird" always depends on who you ask. So ask yourself.

"My partner won't be into that"

This one comes up a lot for male–female couples. Many men with female partners are concerned that the lady in question won't be interested in this sort of play: that she will be grossed out, will think it's weird, or will ask him if he's gay. Well, it's certainly true that some women will react in these ways. But quite a few others will be thrilled to explore prostate play, or will at least be open to trying it. As with any other sexual activity, the best thing to do is talk with your partner about it. (For more tips on opening the conversation for male–female pairings, see chapter 8, Bringing Up the Topic.)

> *"I think my boyfriend was shy about asking me to penetrate him because he had some shame and fear of rejection around his desire for anal play, but I had no inhibitions about it."*

If your girlfriend or wife was the one to suggest prostate play and you're feeling a little nervous about it, we suggest giving it a try. If you discover that you like it, it's one more fun way to have sex. And if you don't enjoy it, at least you were open to checking it out. This makes it a lot easier to bring up your own fantasies and desires when you want to ask her to try them out.

> *"My girlfriend at the time loved having her ass played with and was able to convince me to see how good it could feel. This led to my discovery of how much more intense my orgasm could be when my prostate was being stimulated."*

"My cock is all I need to get off"

For many men, the cock is the star of the show, and that is 100 percent OK. You can keep right on strokin' if that's your inclination. No one is suggesting that you tuck your cock away in the closet and forget about it.

But your cock isn't the only part of your body where you can experience pleasure. There are nerves all over your body just waiting to deliver pleasing sensations to your brain, and there's no reason to ignore them.

Some people seem to think that men should get all their pleasure from their cock: that it somehow makes you more

"I like to know all the spots on my body that can give me pleasure."

masculine if you fixate on the cock to the exclusion of the rest of the body. But we think this is a limiting belief. We are fully in favor of men experiencing more pleasure. Actually, we want *everyone* to have more pleasure.

Maybe it feels good to have your nipples teased. Or maybe you like fingers running through your hair, or having your back scratched. The prostate is just one more part of your body that can feel good to the touch. Lots of men enjoy prostate play in combination with cock play, as a nice enhancer to a hand job or oral sex. Others can enjoy the prostate on its own. Whether or not you include the cock in your prostate play is a simple matter of personal preference.

Exploring new ways of feeling good does not mean that you have to give up old ones. Nor does it mean that you will have to do this every time. You are simply trying something new. If you don't like it, you don't ever have to do it again.

And if you do enjoy it, it can be a tasty new dish to add to your menu of erotic options!

"I had a prostate exam at the doctor's and it didn't feel good at all!"

If your first experience of prostate stimulation happened at the doctor's office, it's not a surprise that it didn't feel good. That's because doctors are trained to make pelvic exams as nonsexual as possible. Of course, they don't want it to feel bad, but they also don't want to raise any questions of sexual harassment with their patients, so they learn how to make it as neutral as they can. Plus, the office may have been chilly, and unless you enjoy doctor–patient role play, the situation was probably about as unerotic as it gets. But don't worry—that doesn't mean you won't like prostate play when it's part of sex.

Think about it like this: plenty of women have had neutral or unpleasant experiences getting pelvic exams at the gynecologist's office, but that doesn't mean they don't enjoy vaginal penetration. The fun kind of prostate play is very different from what happened during your medical exam, so don't let that hold you back.

"Are there health risks?"

Anal penetration involves some risk, though it's pretty easy to minimize it. Rectal tissue is delicate, so it's important to use care and common sense: don't push yourself too hard, never insert an unsafe object, and be mindful that drugs and alcohol may increase your risk of injury by dulling your awareness of pain. For a full list of safety guidelines, see chapter 5, Penetration 101.

That being said, lots of people enjoy anal play very regularly with no long-term ill effects. Some people worry that their sphincter will become loose over time and eventually they won't be able to control their bowel movements, but this is an urban legend. The most common injury resulting from anal penetration is fissures (tiny cuts in the rectal lining), which tend to result from overzealousness. These are usually minor and generally heal on their own.

As for the specific act of massaging the prostate, there is little risk. After all, prostate massage is a routine medical procedure performed by doctors to extract prostatic fluid for testing. In fact, some medical professionals suggest that regular prostate massage can be beneficial to your health by clearing blockages and flushing out potential irritants. For more information regarding the possible health benefits of prostate massage, see chapter 15.

There are certain situations in which prostate massage could be harmful. If you have an acute infection of the prostate, massage may increase the risk of blood poisoning. (See chapter 14, Prostate Health.) However, acute infection comes with serious symptoms of fever and malaise and a very tender prostate that would hurt like the dickens to massage, so it's not likely that you'd want to anyway!

Also, you can get hurt if you are penetrating yourself with an unsafe object or pressing excessively hard. But generally, the main risk is a little bit of bruising, which will result in soreness the following day.

"That all sounds great, but I still don't know how to find my prostate!"

Well, read on, fearless reader! And we will tell you.

2

THE SEXY PROSTATE

"The sensations have varied significantly from session to session. It's difficult to describe—they can vary from significant discomfort, to a feeling of needing to urinate, to no major sensations but an intense feeling of arousal, to complete ecstasy unlike any other sexual experience I've had."

A LITTLE-KNOWN PLEASURE ZONE

The prostate gland is an erogenous zone for a lot of men. It's an area that can create pleasurable, erotic feelings when stimulated. Other erogenous zones include (but are not limited to) the penis, scrotum, clitoris, labia, vagina, nipples, breasts, lips (of the mouth) and the anal area. Many guys have experienced intense pleasure and broader, more powerful orgasms during prostate play. Stimulation of the prostate can trigger an orgasm, and sometimes this happens with prostate play alone, without any cock play.

Although the prostate is not as easy to reach as some of the more readily available erogenous zones, you can find it by inserting a finger about 3–4 inches into the anus and pressing toward the front of the body. The sensation transmits easily through the wall of the rectum to the prostate, which is just on the other side. You can also apply indirect pressure to the prostate through the perineum (the area between the testicles and the anus). According to many men, it takes firm pressure to evoke prostate sensations. Light caresses may feel good, but usually won't bring up the particular sensations that we are talking about.

During arousal, the prostate gland swells, becoming physically larger. Frequently, this swelling is dramatic enough that the giver of a prostate massage can feel the difference with his or her finger. Many men report that they feel the most pleasure when they receive prostate massage at a high level of arousal, when the gland is very engorged. Likewise, too much pressure on an unengorged prostate may feel uninteresting, uncomfortable, or even painful. The swelling increases dramatically just before ejaculation, and many men can take very firm pressure leading up to and during climax.

It may come as a surprise to hear that the prostate can be an erogenous zone. Many men have never heard of the prostate, except in relation to cancer and uncomfortable rectal exams at the doctor's office. Outside the gay community and other sexual subcultures, male-receptive anal penetration is often considered taboo, so even though lots of men of all sexual orientations play with their prostate with a partner or during masturbation, many of them are not talking about it openly. As a result, the erotic nature of the prostate is not widely acknowledged in mainstream culture. We think this is a pity. However, this is changing as more and more male–female pairs are learning about and trying out this kind of play.

YOUR MILEAGE MAY VARY

Hearing descriptions of the erogenous nature of the prostate may be helpful when you are first trying prostate play. It can be exciting to know what the possibilities are. And if your first few tries don't work out the way you had hoped, it can be encouraging to hear other people's positive experiences.

However, any description you read about how prostate play feels is necessarily about how it feels *to someone else*. With prostate play, or any other kind of sex, what's most important is how it feels *to you*. And the only way to find out how it feels to you is to try it for yourself, and then experiment and practice.

Someone else's description may not match what you feel. It might simply be that you are using different words to describe a similar feeling. For example, one guy may describe a swollen, engorged prostate as feeling "full" while another might say it feels "heavy." There is a limit to how well a subjective sensation can be translated into words.

Also, with any kind of sexual experience, tastes differ. What you like won't work for everyone, and what someone else enjoys might not work for you. And on top of that, preferences change over time. Don't worry if your experiences are different from someone else's—this is normal! Everyone is different, and it doesn't mean that there's something wrong with you if the things we describe don't work for you right away, or ever.

For some men, playing with their prostate feels good the very first time, while others may not feel pleasure right away. The prostate may be tender for the first few experiences, and for those who are new to anal penetration, there may be some discomfort associated with it. This tends to decrease with practice as the prostate and anus grow accustomed to being stimulated, and it is possible for someone who doesn't feel much pleasure at first to come to like it if he tries it again at a later time.

Initially, pressure on this area is unfamiliar and might feel very strange. The area may feel numb, or produce a tingling sensation. It is also very common to say that it makes you feel like you have to pee. If the stimulation continues, these feelings often give way to pleasure. Men have described the feelings of pleasure as being "almost unbearably intense" and "excruciatingly good."

"At first it made me feel like I had to pee and now I am not sure I can describe it other than 'amazing.'"

"[I feel] discomfort—at first, with some feeling like I need to pee, but then it just starts [to] accentuate the feelings from my cock and anal sphincter."

"Sort of a cross between the need to urinate and come."

"At first, the pressure is foreign and made me worried that I might need to use the restroom. There are times when the pressure can make my bladder feel very full. I've learned that this is just normal for me so I'm able to relax and not worry about the sensation if it occurs (which it doesn't very often)."

"Originally it felt utterly alien and brought neither pleasure nor discomfort. Now I have had anal orgasms from this."

A UNIQUE SENSATION

Cock play and prostate play can both be intensely pleasurable, and many men are struck by how distinctly different these two sensations feel. The way it feels to touch the head of the cock is quite different from the way it feels to contact the prostate. They have both have been described as "more intense" in their own way.

Sensations from cock stimulation are often described as "focused," "localized," or "specific to one area," and also as "external" and "superficial." Typically, the sensations are concentrated in the penis (especially at the head) and are very intensely felt in that area.

By comparison, prostate stimulation tends to feel "dull," "diffuse," and "less sharp." It is also described as "broader" and "more encompassing" of a larger area. The stimulation feels "internal" and seems to "radiate from within" and "extend outward," having an effect on other parts of the genitals, the pelvis, or the whole body.

> *"Prostate stimulation can be otherworldly, like you are not sure where the pleasure is coming from. Penis stimulation, now, while still nice, is more to the point."*
>
> *"Totally different. [Prostate stimulation feels] duller and less intense in the sense of concentrated excitement, but very powerful and intense in a more full-body experience way."*
>
> *"It is a deeper, fuller, more encompassing pleasure, radiating from within the body instead of feeling like external stimulation."*
>
> *"Penile stimulation is about certain external 'hot spots,' while prostate stimulation is all internal."*

In our survey, almost every part of the body was named as an area to which sensations could radiate during prostate massage. However, certain parts were emphasized, especially the penis (head, shaft, and base), the testicles, the anus, and the pelvic area generally. There may be a "noticeable increase in strength of erection and blood flow," and feelings of "warmth," "fullness," "swelling," "pulsing," or "throbbing" in the specific areas of the genitals, or the whole genital region.

> *"It makes my ass and cock tingle in the most delicious way that gets me harder than any other stimulation."*
>
> *"Stroking my prostate feels like some invisible hand is also stroking my cock and balls in close synchronization."*
>
> *"The sensation often seems to radiate into the testes and base of the penis, sometimes making the head throb. Sometimes I get shivers."*
>
> *"[It] feels like the head of my penis is going to explode, feels really incredible. My entire penis pulses."*
>
> *"My penis is much more sensitive when my prostate is being stimulated."*

A number of men reported that the radiating sensations throughout the pelvic area brought up a feeling of unification of the genitals. One man responded to the question "How is the sensation of prostate stimulation different from that of penis stimulation?" by saying, "It isn't. It makes it feel like my cock starts at my ass."

> "It brings together all the erogenous zones into one 'total' pleasure zone, connecting penis stimulation with anal stimulation."
>
> "It is a deeper, more intense sensation that feels like your penis is being stimulated from behind...from its origin inside."
>
> "Slow in-and-out stimulation feels like a total release and total gathering of my entire pelvic/anal regions."

A number of men also emphasized that sensations are felt radiating "everywhere, the whole body." Some described it as "tingling," "shivers," or "a warm feeling all over."

> "[I feel an] all-over bodily sensation, a sense of my whole body being connected to that spot. [I feel it as] sexual pleasure to the whole penis, and as a glowing, good feeling in my whole body."

PROSTATE PLEASURE
FOR TRANSGENDER WOMEN

Though this book is addressed to men, it's important to note that transgender women also have a prostate. Transgender women are persons who were assigned a male gender at birth but identify as female. They might choose to take a variety of steps to bring their gender identity and their body into closer alignment, such as taking hormones and surgery.

The transgender women we've heard from have had varying experiences with prostate play, ranging from "I don't do it at all" to "I enjoy it a lot!" Some women may call it "my prostate," while others prefer to call it "my G-spot" or use other terms.

One woman who enjoys prostate play shared her experience with us: "I absolutely love to have my prostate rubbed like a genie bottle or a turntable. It makes me feel like I'm on the edge of a cliff and my toes are curling and squeezing the last of the soil and I couldn't give a shit if I fell. Just pure bliss."

Another woman offered a very different perspective: "I am quick to say I don't see my prostate as a pleasurable entity. It might be. I am not aware of it. I see it more as a remnant of male stuff I am not interested in. I don't hate it or anything. It is just one more thing I have reminding me of all that 'stuff.' If I am sexually excited I don't have a form of 'Oh, that's my prostate' or anything. If I did it would creep me out. No, I'll just go on blissfully ignorant to any contribution to pleasure my prostate provides. Serious buzzkill comes to mind."

Because people can have such different thoughts and feelings about prostate play, it's always best to ask instead of trying to guess. In our view, that's good advice about any kind of sex!

Since different women make different choices regarding genital realignment surgery, there are various possibilities when it comes to P-spot play. Those who have not had genital surgery can locate it using the same techniques that work on cisgender men. Transgender women who choose genital surgery may stimulate it in a different way, depending on the exact procedure used. One method positions the vaginal canal behind the prostate, which puts the prostate in the general location of the G-spot in cisgender women. However, the vaginal canal will often be angled more sharply, depending on each person's individual anatomy. As a result, some transgender women will not need as much tilt in their hips or as curved a toy to reach the prostate.

Also, many take hormones to feminize the body, and this may have an effect on prostate play as well. These hormones cause the prostate to shrink, which may make it more difficult to locate. At this time, there aren't any studies that explore prostate sensitivity, but some transgender women report that after taking hormones for a while they stop ejaculating, and that the feeling of the orgasm is different. One woman describes her experience: "I must say that having my prostate stimulated does not make me come immediately the way it did before hormones and testosterone blockers. Now it is more of a build up and release of energy, with or without ejaculation."

Because someone's erotic sensations from prostate stimulation may shift, your best bet is to ask what their desires and preferences are. The answers will vary from person to person and may shift over time, so don't assume that what a previous partner enjoyed will work for a new one. It's also a good idea to ask a transgender woman her preferred language for talking about this kind of play: prostate play, G-spot, or something else. Let her choices around this guide your actions.

PROSTATE ORGASM

In addition to feeling really good, prostate stimulation can trigger an orgasm. In some cases, this happens almost immediately. Many men say that they sometimes feel "like I'm about to come" nearly instantly after the prostate is touched, and sometimes *do* actually come right away. This is especially common among men who are new to the stimulation. The pleasure is so sudden and unexpected that they may go right over the edge.

> *"When my prostate is stimulated, I sometimes feel as if I am going to climax immediately (and sometimes do)."*
>
> *"It feels like I am being physically pushed toward ejaculation."*
>
> *"[I] have ejaculated instantly after prostate contact."*

Prostate stimulation can trigger an ejaculatory orgasm with or without simultaneous cock stimulation, though it is much more common when both of these areas are pleasured at the same time. (Prostate stimulation can trigger nonejaculatory orgasms as well—more on that below.) Also, some find that prostate massage makes it easier to come more quickly during penis stimulation, and to come without being fully erect.

> *"I have never actually come until I stimulate my penis, even if it is just one quick stroke."*
>
> *"I can't orgasm from just prostate stimulation like some. I need to masturbate in unison."*
>
> *"I've never ejaculated solely from prostate stimulation, but it makes it possible to orgasm after only a few strokes of the penis. Prostate stimulation also makes it easier to ejaculate without the penis being fully erect."*

When prostate massage leads to an ejaculatory orgasm without cock stimulation, it is sometimes referred to as "milking the prostate." However, this term is also sometimes used to mean prostate massage generally, since massage stimulates the release of prostatic fluid. It is common for fluid to run from the tip of the cock, ranging from a few drops to an abundant flow, even without ejaculation.

Orgasms from prostate massage alone are often described as coming on very suddenly and unexpectedly. It is common for those who have had this experience to say that it happened only once or twice, and that they have found it difficult to replicate the experience intentionally.

> "[It] caught me by surprise. Intensity went from 3 to 10 in seconds. Has only happened twice."
>
> "THAT was intense and pleasurable, but we haven't figured out how to repeat it."

Just as many men report that prostate sensations feel different from cock sensations, orgasms that involve prostate stimulation (with or without ejaculation) often feel different from those that come from cock stimulation alone. The differences between the two types of orgasm mirror the differences between the sensations generally. According to some men's descriptions, the orgasm is felt "deeper" in the body, and the prostate is felt to be the trigger of the orgasm, the place where the orgasm originates.

"Oftentimes the prostate triggers the orgasm and it usually feels deeper."

"It feels like it comes from the base of the penis rather than the tip."

"Rather than the pressure (for lack of a better word) building up in the tip of the penis, it builds up in the base."

"They begin with a deeper feeling like a wave that rolls up and overwhelms me."

Penis-focused orgasms tend to feel localized. The sensation is powerful and very pleasurable, but it is centered in a limited, local area—namely, the area of the genitals and particularly the cock. Prostate-focused orgasms, on the other hand, often feel broader and more diffuse, and are reported to last longer. The sensation may be felt in larger portions of the genital area, the pelvis, and even the whole body (full-body orgasm).

"It is the gateway to full-body orgasm."

"I often have a whole body orgasm, a kind of ripple through and a sense of being out of my body."

"The orgasm is usually far more intense. The orgasm seems to radiate all over my body instead of being localized."

"It seems bigger, like I'm opened up inside and can contain more pleasure, if that makes sense."

FULL-BODY ORGASM

Full-body orgasms are known by many names, including Tantric orgasm, implosive orgasm, and energy orgasm. People who have experienced one describe it as taking the pleasure sensation that you feel during orgasm and spreading it out through the body, drawing it to other parts so that you feel orgasmic sensations not just in the genitals, but all over.

Somraj Pokras and Jeffre TallTrees, authors of the e-book *Tantric Male Multiple G-spot Orgasm*, put it this way: "When Kundalini energy streams throughout your body, it's as if every cell is climaxing. Yes, those same ecstatic vibrations you normally feel in your jewels during an explosion, you feel them everywhere." (For an explanation of Kundalini energy, see the sidebar "The Root Chakra" in chapter 3.)

Because prostate sensations already tend to feel "broader," many men find that prostate play lends itself very well to spreading the sensation beyond the genital area. This is a technique that may require a lot of practice, but if you'd like to learn it, check out the e-book mentioned above, or Mantak Chia's guide to multiple orgasms.

The orgasm is often described as more intense than an orgasm that doesn't involve prostate stimulation. There may also be a sense of releasing control.

> "My orgasms are always much stronger, by a factor of three or four times at least."

> "The orgasms of prostate play combined with penile stimulation tend to be stronger and more intense than with penile stimulation alone."

"It comes from the inside, it's totally different in that I cannot control anything, I really feel that I need to relinquish control totally."

Many men say that ejaculation during prostate play feels "more powerful," "forceful," or "explosive," with stronger contractions, and the ejaculation/orgasm tends to last longer. There is often quite a lot of fluid dripping prior to ejaculation, and possibly a larger-than-average volume of semen. This is great fun for those who eroticize sex fluids and appreciate large quantities.

When the prostate is massaged during ejaculation, the fluid may flow out rather than shoot out. This may be a downer for fans of more dramatic, projectile ejaculations. (If you're in this boat, just arrange yourself in a facedown position so that gravity is on your side!)

"Extremely intense. More feelings of pleasure from the ejaculation than without prostate stimulation. And a feeling of way more ejaculate."

"My orgasms are larger and the ejaculation pressure is much greater."

"Such orgasms are very strong and tend to produce much more semen... The pulses are very strong, like all the organs are pumping as hard as possible."

"The ejaculation is less of a spurt and goes on for longer."

Orgasms that occur during prostate stimulation are also associated with stronger and more long-lasting after-effects.

"It doesn't seem to end as fast, or be the cliff of enjoyment that occurs after non-prostate stimulation orgasm."

"Following a session of fisting, PC contractions elicit waves of pleasure for as much as a few hours while my prostate is still hypersensitized."

"I find that pleasurable sensations continue much longer than after a 'normal' orgasm, both in terms of the prostate itself and a heightened sense of postcoital release and relaxation."

LINGERING ON THE BRINK

We mentioned that when the prostate is contacted, sometimes it feels like you're about to come right away, and sometimes men *do* come almost instantly. However, it is also possible to stay with that feeling of being about to come without actually going over the edge and ejaculating.

In fact, even though prostate massage can bring you so quickly to the verge of orgasm/ejaculation, many men say that they find it easier to hold off from ejaculating with prostate play than during penile stimulation. This is particularly true if you are judicious about how much you stimulate the cock at the same time: "Too much penis stimulation with prostate stimulation will make me orgasm too quickly every time," one respondent said.

"The sensation is less intensely pleasurable, but also less urgent; it is easier to enjoy it in its own right without feeling compelled to continue to orgasm."

"[It feels] like it is causing me to and preventing me from orgasm at the same time."

> *"It's very difficult for me to ejaculate from anal play alone—which is something I really like about it, as it can lengthen the experience and make the entire session much more satisfying."*

If you are able to resist the impulse to ejaculate, you can linger in that "preorgasmic" feeling. Prostate play can give you that feeling of impending orgasm for an extended period of time, instead of just a few moments before ejaculation, as with a typical ejaculatory orgasm. The duration ranges from many minutes to hours. There is a sense that the feeling "can be perpetuated basically indefinitely."

> *"Prostate stimulation gives me a feeling like no other, almost euphoric, constantly on the verge of coming."*
>
> *"The sensation is very similar [to] the sensation I feel right before I have an orgasm. The best thing about it is that this sensation can be prolonged for long periods of time rather than just the fleeting seconds prior to the orgasm itself."*
>
> *"The few moments before ejaculation are intense, and prostate play increases the length of time that occurs."*
>
> *"It is a feeling I want to last. It's hard to stop prostate stimulation because it is so good. It's not about wanting the release of orgasm. It is a deeper gratification."*
>
> *"Sometimes having my penis stimulated and ejaculating is just a way to stop."*

In this way, prostate stimulation can take on a different arousal pattern than cock stimulation. Penis stimulation typically (but not always) builds up to the brink of ejaculatory orgasm. You spend a few moments in the preorgasmic state, and then you go over the edge, ejaculate, and enter a refractory period (of varying duration) during which you can't become erect, have an orgasm, or ejaculate again. With prostate stimulation, it is possible to jump very quickly to the brink of orgasm, but then you can stay in that state for a very long time.

To put this another way, let's say that on a scale of zero to 10, zero is a completely unaroused state and 10 is the peak of orgasm. During cock stimulation, the arousal level often hits a plateau, though there may be peaks and valleys along the way. When orgasm happens, it jumps up to 8, 9, and 10 in a very short time frame, then drops rapidly to zero.

With prostate play, if you aren't rushing yourself or causing pain during penetration, there will generally be some arousal already happening, either from simultaneous cock stimulation or at least from stimulation of the sensitive nerves of the anus, so you're probably at least in the 3 to 5 range, if not higher. Once the gland is contacted, the arousal can jump quite suddenly to an 8, but then it can hover around that level for a much longer time. Some say this happens almost immediately, while others say that it may take them a little while to get there, but the experience of hovering at that level is quite common.

Some men say that while lingering on the brink they experience intermittent and repeated peaks of intensity. Some describe this as an orgasm (a 10!), while others seem to think of it as "orgasmic" but not quite an orgasm. However, the experience is described very similarly by those who say it's an orgasm and those who don't call it that, so it's possible that they are actually talking about the same thing. It is typical to describe it as a wave that crashes over you. After these peaks, the arousal level can return to an 8 and hover there again until the stimulation stops or ejaculation ushers in the refractory period.

> *"A penile orgasm is very much about the need to come and is centered in that area. You just work your penis and the pressure builds, then you pop... P-spot orgasm is much more like a wave crashing down on you. When it hits, you feel it over all of your body. The P-spot orgasm is something that does not pop. [It is] more like waves that run across your body one after another."*

> *"The sensations from prostate stimulation [can] be as intensely pleasurable as an orgasm, though not following the same kind of pattern (a huge wave of pleasure which then slowly peters out). It is more like repeated spikes of orgasmic pleasure with no real resolution."*

> *"Repeated stimulation (in–out motions or occasionally vibrations) can create incredibly pleasurable sensations that do not conform to the standard arousal pattern (excitement, plateau, orgasm, resolution). Instead, it tends to deliver pleasurable sensations that are not linear and are more stochastic in nature, seeming to never reach a single, conclusive peak."*

> *"The orgasm involves entire body convulsions which are extremely pleasurable. It lasts approximately 3 minutes per orgasm and the orgasms tend to come in waves, with a great amount of precum but little or no ejaculate."*

MULTIPLE ORGASMS

Many people use the terms *orgasm* and *ejaculation* interchangeably, at least when talking about men's sexual responses. Although orgasm and ejaculation often happen at the same time, or at least close together, they are not the same thing. Ejaculation is the emission and expulsion of semen, while orgasm is the experience of pleasurable release. In terms of the nervous system, ejaculation is a spinal cord reflex, whereas orgasm happens in the cerebral cortex of the brain.

Because ejaculation and orgasm are two distinct processes, it is possible to have one without the other. If you've ever reached the "point of no return" during sex or masturbation and the motion was interrupted, you may have discovered that it is possible to ejaculate without the usual pleasure of orgasm. One fellow told us, "Once, I ejaculated from prostate stimulation alone without experiencing orgasm. That was boring."

Luckily, it goes the other way too: you can also have an orgasm without ejaculating, which means that it is possible for men to have multiple orgasms. Because ejaculation causes a latency period of at least a few minutes (sometimes a lot longer) during which you can't ejaculate again, usually an ejaculatory orgasm means no more orgasms for a while. But if you learn to orgasm without ejaculating, there is no latency period and you can keep going! (If you'd like to learn how to be multiorgasmic, see the Resources at the back of the book for some guides that we recommend.)

Once you learn to separate orgasm from ejaculation, it is possible to have as many as eight or more orgasms during a prolonged session. Many men who practice this technique have a series of nonejaculatory orgasms and then wrap it up with an ejaculatory one. Or you might choose not to ejaculate at all, in the Taoist tradition of withholding ejaculation.

If you're interested in exploring multiple orgasm techniques, you'll want to get your PC muscle in shape. Actually, that's a good idea whether your agenda includes multiple orgasms or not. Check out chapter 6, Searching for the "Magic Button," for info.

Some men say that ending the session with ejaculation feels more intense than ejaculating from penis stimulation alone, though some men report that it can actually feel less intense, or only slightly more intense than usual. However, they may feel that the prolonged experience of "lingering on the brink" is intense enough to make that worthwhile. And it can even vary from one session to another, for the same guy.

> *"Often I find that the penile sensations during orgasm are reduced by prostate stimulation, though paradoxically the sensations leading up to orgasm are dramatically more intense. The orgasmic pleasure itself tends to be less localized to any particular area of my body and can range from less intense than my average penile orgasm to significantly more intense."*
>
> *"When I do reach orgasm, the orgasm can be extremely strong or it can end up being weak, even if I was really excited to begin with. In those cases, the prostate stimulation became an end in itself, and the main experience of pleasure."*

THE PROSTATE'S ROLE IN ANAL PLEASURE

Men who enjoy prostate sensation often consider it to be the main event when it comes to anal penetration. It can be a major contributor to the pleasure of being penetrated, and for some, it's the whole point. However, the prostate is not the only reason why anal play can feel good for a man—there are many highly sensitive nerve endings at the anal opening, and lots of men enjoy the feeling of having the rectum filled up as well.

Some men feel prostate sensations as distinct among the other pleasurable sensations of anal penetration. One fellow described his experience: "Anal pleasure is the general feeling of fullness. The prostate is more like hitting that special button. Anal pleasure is mostly made by the sensation of being filled up and stretched out and penetrated. And prostate play involves a very special set of nerves. They coincide but it's a whole different frequency. When it suddenly hits, there's an 'ooh!' Of course, it's tricky when that 'ooh' happens not to tense up and lose it, but to ride out that sensation."

Others don't notice prostate sensations as distinct: "For me, anal penetration feels good and feels better than external anal stimulation. Based on my reading I believe that the prostate accounts for much of that [...] though frankly apart from reading I don't know that I would have concluded that there was a special spot corresponding to the prostate that was especially pleasurable."

In cases like this it is unclear whether the person is actually feeling his prostate but doesn't sense it as distinct from other pleasurable sensations, or is just not tuning in to his prostate (in the same way that a woman can have her vagina penetrated but not feel G-spot sensations).

However, there are some instances where it is fairly clear that a man has stimulated the area of the prostate during penetration, because he describes some of the other hallmarks of prostate stimulation (particularly needing to pee), but he doesn't like it. Some of these men simply don't enjoy anal penetration at all. However, there are those who say they enjoy anal penetration very much but applying pressure to the prostate just doesn't feel good. Or, they may say they can enjoy a slight grazing of the prostate during penetration, but focused pressure, as with a prostate massage, feels "overwhelming."

> "I enjoy anal play, I wanted to try this. I actually don't enjoy it, it's a weird pressure and inhibits my orgasms... I generally try to avoid it and just have the anal without the pressure."

> "I did not enjoy the feeling of pressure in my abdomen. This feeling has been prevalent throughout my anal play experiments, and I've not been able to derive pleasure from the stimulation."

> "Counterintuitively, I find that indirect prostate stimulation sometimes produces a more intense orgasm than direct prostate stimulation. For example, inserting a finger less than 1 inch and pressing inward against the walls of the inner sphincter often produces very sharp, explosive pleasure on the prostate itself during orgasm. Conversely, inserting a finger [deeper] to directly massage the prostate often generates a more vague, diffuse, 'uninspired' orgasm."

OTHER REASONS TO ENJOY PROSTATE STIMULATION

In addition to all the delicious sensations we have described, there are a number of other reasons why men enjoy prostate stimulation. Many said that they love the variety that it brings to their sex life. Also, if the man is usually on the giving end of penetration, the role reversal can be a nice change as well as a psychological turn-on.

> *"It gives me variety to add to masturbation."*
>
> *"The prospect of a new type of pleasure, as well as the exploration of my body and sexuality, is what made me interested in trying it."*
>
> *"I enjoy exploring my body and pleasuring myself."*
>
> *"It feels great and offers me a realm of sexual exploration outside of the limited palette that men are often stuck with."*
>
> *"I like the sense of role reversal, with my wife penetrating me."*
>
> *"It makes me feel like my partner is interested in giving me pleasure, and that makes me feel desired and sexy."*
>
> *"It is very erotic—being able to relax and have my partner take care of me."*
>
> *"It's nice to not be 'in charge.'"*

Others expressed appreciation for the "naughty" factor. Because of the widespread idea that men are not supposed to receive, let alone enjoy, penetration, it can feel like you are doing something "forbidden," and that can add a major psychological charge. The common notion that penetration is an act of dominance opens the door to fantasies of dominance and submission for those who enjoy that kind of role play.

"It's the secret spot and secrets can be sweet."

"The physical sensation is great, as well as the psychological stimulation of doing something 'naughty.'"

"We incorporate it into our BDSM play and it's erotic because she dominates me with this play."

"The idea of being dominated and penetrated is an incredibly sexy one to me."

Others emphasize the deep feelings of intimacy that they experience when they open up (literally and figuratively) to their partner. Because of the vulnerability associated with anal penetration, it takes a great deal of trust in your partner to let them play with that part of your body. Experiencing that trust can make you feel closer.

"[For me] it's definitely not because it's 'forbidden' or 'naughty.' It feels very intimate. The sensation of penetration, having someone inside you, has an unparalleled sense of erotic closeness."

"The psychological part is enjoying being fucked, of opening my body to another. Feeling him/her inside me."

"I enjoy it because my butt is the most sensitive part of my body, and also where I feel the greatest amount of vulnerability with a partner—meaning I get to feel the trust with a partner enough to fully let go of my inhibitions, emotionally, and give myself to another. Feels very empowering, plus the sensations are fantastic."

"It takes a lot of trust to let someone play with you that way. The level of openness and trust is erotic."

With all these different experiences, thoughts, and feelings about prostate play, there are many possibilities for you to explore. Part of what makes it so exciting is that you get to find out how it will work for you!

3

WHAT IS THE PROSTATE?

"When it comes to sex we tend to focus mainly on the penis, but sexual stimulation actually involves many different parts of our bodies working together to create pleasurable sensations."

—MICHAEL THOMAS FORD

The prostate gland is a part of the male sexual and reproductive anatomy. It is responsible for making prostatic fluid, one of the main components of semen. The rest of the fluid that makes up semen is produced by the seminal vesicles, the bulbourethral (aka Cowper's) glands, and the testes/ epididymis. Estimates of the proportions of these fluids vary widely, but most agree that the contributions of the testes/

epididymis (which provide the actual sperm) and the bulbo-urethral glands make up a relatively small portion of the total semen volume, while the bulk of it comes from the prostate and seminal vesicles.

PROSTATE ANATOMY

The most common way people describe the prostate gland is to compare it to a walnut. This is a good image to convey its size and shape, particularly for a young man. (The prostate tends to grow with age.) But as far as texture is concerned, the prostate is not hard and dry like a walnut, so we enjoy the alternative comparison suggested in *Dr. Peter Scardino's Prostate Book*: "a small plum, with its spongy, fluid-filled interior and soft skin."[1] This is a more palatable image for the prostate

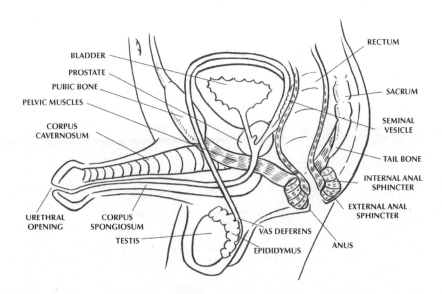

Illustration 1. Male Anatomy

in terms of texture, and it is close in shape as well. Now, for that small plum to be the size of the prostate of a young man, it would need, in fact, to be a *walnut-sized* plum—very small indeed. For men whose prostate has grown with age (due to BPH or cancer), "a larger and sometimes more irregular plum would serve as a reasonable surrogate image."[2]

So imagine that small plum, only instead of a pit in the center, imagine a straw running through it vertically. That's the urethra, which starts at the bottom of the bladder, passes through the prostate, and then curves forward to run along the length of the penis. The prostate sits directly beneath the bladder and above the bulb of the penis (separated by a layer of muscle—the external urethral sphincter). It is located centrally in the pelvis, behind the pubic bone and in front of the rectum.

SHALL I COMPARE THEE TO A WALNUT?

One fellow we interviewed said that each time he looks for the prostate, he thinks to himself, OK, find the walnut. The walnut is the quintessential image people use to convey the general size and shape of the prostate, but you could compare it to a number of other things too. To broaden the options a bit, here are some other images and terms we have encountered:

a chestnut	"his special spot"
an avocado seed	"the grand gland"
a golf ball	"that round little bulge"
"the bulb"	"the male Sacred Gate"[3]
"my knob"	a "slightly squishy
"his sweet spot"	super-bounce ball"

Remember that we said the prostate was a gland? A gland is an organ of the body that produces a substance. Well, the prostate is also made up of glands: the individual, microscopic glands (called *acini*) which are tiny factories for fluid production. It's a bit confusing, because the term *gland* applies to both the individual glands and the collective organ that they form. Think of it as a whole lot of tiny water balloons all interconnected and encased in one large water balloon.

During arousal, the tiny, microscopic *acini* that make up the glandular tissue of the prostate are busily producing fluid. This makes the prostate swell as all those little water balloons fill up. Increased blood flow to the area may contribute to swelling as well. Some men who are very tuned in to their prostate can sense this swelling as a feeling of fullness at the base of the cock. It is often so dramatic that you can feel the difference with your finger during a prostate massage. As the prostate swells up and expands, its shape changes, becoming more rounded, and a larger portion of the prostate can be felt bulging against the rectal wall, making it easier to locate with a finger.

Each of the *acini* is connected to a channel called a *duct* which opens into the prostatic urethra (the portion of the urethra that runs through the prostate). During ejaculation, involuntary smooth muscles within the prostate contract rhythmically, squeezing the prostatic fluid out of the glands, through the ducts, and into the prostatic urethra.

PHASES OF EJACULATION

Ejaculation happens in two phases: emission and ejaculation.[4] (To avoid confusion, the latter is sometimes called "expulsion.") During the first phase, emission, the prostate and other sex glands emit (release) their various contributions to the semen. These fluids are all pumped into the prostatic urethra.

Once the emission phase has started and the fluids have begun to be pumped into the prostatic urethra, the second phase, expulsion, occurs, during which the fluids are sent rushing through the urethra and out the tip of the cock.

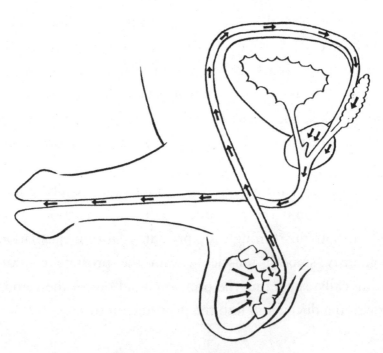

Illustration 2. Course of Sperm

COURSE OF SPERM

Sperm are manufactured in the testes, then stored in two epididymides (the singular is *epididymis*) that sit on top of the testicles like little hats. During the first phase of ejaculation, the sperm are released from both epididymides and sent up through the vas deferens: two tubes (one on each side) that rise from the scrotum and up into the body. The tubes rise toward the front of the body, then loop around to the backside of the prostate, where they widen into the ejaculatory ducts. The ejaculatory ducts enter the back of the prostate and lead into the prostatic urethra. They carry the sperm as well as the fluid from the seminal vesicles, a pair of glands extending out from the back of the prostate like a pair of wings. Meanwhile, the prostatic fluid is sent into the prostatic urethra, so that all these fluids can be expelled through the tip of the cock.

THE MALE G-SPOT?

"One cannot help but be struck by the similarity between descriptions of prostate stimulation and reports from women upon discovering their G spot."

—ALICE KAHN LADAS, BEVERLY WHIPPLE, AND JOHN D. PERRY

The "male G-spot" is a name that more and more people are using for the prostate, especially when talking about its erotic potential. This has given rise to another term, the *P-spot*. Use of these names is especially common among sex educators and sexuality product retailers, though many people outside these communities also enjoy the idea of a male G-spot. There are a few reasons for thinking of the prostate as the male G-spot, which we will explain. But first, what is the G-spot?

In 1982, Ladas et al. published the bestselling book *The G Spot and Other Recent Discoveries about Human Sexuality*, bringing this erogenous zone into widespread (contemporary) public awareness. They described the G-spot as a "sensitive area" that is usually located "directly behind the pubic bone within the front wall of the vagina ... along the course of the urethra ... and near the neck of the bladder, where it connects to the urethra."[5] They noted that this area is responsive to deep pressure, swells when stimulated, and that some women can reach orgasm through the stimulation.

They also describe "female ejaculation"—the release of a small amount of fluid from the urethra that sometimes occurs during G-spot stimulation. They cite the suggestion, previously offered by J. Lowndes Sevely and J.W. Bennett (and others before them), that some women ejaculate and that the expelled fluid comes from the female prostate.[6]

There is still some disagreement regarding female ejaculation, but for our purposes what is important is that female ejaculation was often observed to occur during G-spot stimulation (though it can occur at other times as well), and therefore the glandular tissue of the female prostate was suggested as the source of the expelled fluid. This link between the female prostate and the G-spot was further strengthened by the fact that this glandular tissue was in the right location to be stimulated during G-spot play, and offered an explanation for the swelling that was observed. So, because of these perceived links, many people began to talk of the G-spot as if it *were* the female prostate.[7]

WHAT IS THE FEMALE PROSTATE?

As described above, the male prostate encircles the urethra below the bladder and is made up of glands and ducts that empty into the urethra. Females also have glands and ducts that surround and empty into the urethra. This glandular tissue has been called the paraurethral glands or Skene's glands, but it is increasingly being called the "female prostate," since this tissue is homologous to the prostate in the male.

What does it mean that the male and female prostate are *homologous*? It means that they are formed from the same tissue in an embryo. In the early stages of pregnancy all human embryos have the same blueprint anatomy, regardless of their future sex. The genetic sex is already determined by chromosomes, but for the first several weeks all embryos have the same basic structures with the potential to develop into different genitals, depending on fetal development.

Since the sex organs develop from the same template, the resulting forms have many similarities. This is the meaning of *homology*. Every part of the male and female sex organs corresponds to a *homologue* in the other sex. For example, the testes and the ovaries are homologous. Likewise, it is widely agreed that the male and female prostate are homologous.

Although the female prostate is commonly believed to be the female G-spot (that is to say, many believe that it is the anatomic structure responsible for G-spot sensations), this has not been established scientifically. The trouble is, this glandular tissue has not been shown to contain the types of nerve endings or the density of nerve endings that are usually found in an area of sensitive tissue.[8] There is still plenty of controversy over exactly how the application of pressure to the area known as the G-spot leads to the sensations that women report, given that "no appropriate structure and innervation have been clearly demonstrated in this pleasurable vaginal area."[9]

Back to the (male) prostate. In *The G-spot*, Ladas et al. point out that "men also have a pleasurable area located, like the G spot, around the urethra at the neck of the bladder. It is known as the prostate gland."[10] They also point out that descriptions of how it feels to stimulate this area are very similar to descriptions of G-spot stimulation.[11]

SIMILARITIES BETWEEN PROSTATE AND G-SPOT STIMULATION AND SENSATION

- Both can be stimulated by reaching a short distance inside the body—about 2–3 inches vaginally for the G-spot, and about 3–4 inches anally for the prostate—and pressing through the front (anterior) wall.

- Both tend to respond to the same kinds of strokes. Most people who enjoy this stimulation find that they need deep pressure, not light caresses, to feel these sensations.

- Stimulation of both may result, initially, in a feeling like the need to urinate.

- For both, this stimulation is much more likely to feel pleasurable if arousal is high before it begins.

- Stimulation of both may result in orgasm, with or without simultaneous stimulation of the external areas of the penis/clitoris.

- Prostate and G-spot orgasms are often described as being subjectively different from orgasms that result from stimulation of the glans of the penis/clitoris (respectively). They reportedly feel "broader" and more "full-bodied" when compared to the more "local" or "focused" sensation of a penis/clitoris-induced orgasm.

- Prostate- and G-spot-induced orgasms are described as being felt "deeper" in the body, without the usual contractions of the pelvic floor muscles that occur with penis/clitoris-induced orgasms, though there may be contractions of deeper pelvic muscles.

So there are a few reasons why people talk about the prostate as the "male G-spot"—some of them valid, some maybe not. Calling the prostate the "male G-spot" or the P-spot highlights the fact that men, too, have a very powerful internal pleasure button to be explored, and that for men and women it's located in the same basic area, responds to the same kinds of stimulation, and feels very similar. This suggests that whatever is going on neurologically, it is the same for both.

In addition, people have called the male prostate the "male G-spot" because they believed the female prostate was the female G-spot. However, since it's not clear that the female prostate is responsible for female G-spot sensations, some sex experts disagree with this terminology.

ABOUT NERVES

At this point, we'd like to make a few observations about nerves. The body has different neural systems that serve different functions. The sensory/motor system controls voluntary, conscious activity. Most of the sensory receptors of the body are a part of the sensory/motor system. Different kinds of sensory receptors pick up different kinds of stimuli. When a sensory receptor picks up a stimulus to which it is sensitive (has the capacity to register), it sends a signal to the brain—or to the spinal cord, in the case of a spinal cord reflex. When the brain receives the signal, it can interpret the sensation as pleasurable or otherwise. The pudendal nerve, which innervates the skin of the penis (and also the perineum and anus), is part of the sensory/motor system and has plenty of sensory receptors that send signals to the brain/spinal cord.

There is also the autonomic nervous system, which controls involuntary (and often unconscious) functions of the body, such as blood pressure, breathing rate, and perspiration. It also controls arousal and ejaculation. The pelvic plexus, which innervates the prostate gland, is part of the autonomic nervous system. The portion of the pelvic plexus that innervates the prostate is called the prostatic plexus. The nerves of the prostatic plexus serve important functions in emission and ejaculation. Also, some of the nerves in the prostatic plexus continue to the corpora cavernosa of the penis and are responsible for erection.

The prostatic plexus contains some limited sensory receptors that travel with the autonomic nerves, but not many, and these receptors are not able to pick up a wide range of sensation. So we find ourselves with the same question as with the female G-spot: if the male prostate does not have the kinds of sensory receptors that would allow an area to be "sensitive" and to send lots of sensory input to the brain for the brain to interpret as pleasurable, can the prostate really be said to be the source of the good feelings that men experience during prostate massage?

Myrtle Wilhite MD says no: "Massaging the gland itself (while it has health benefits of pushing some fluid out) does not lead to sexual arousal." She suggests that what is really happening is that the autonomic nerves of the prostatic plexus are being massaged—and the impact of this massage is not mediated by sensory receptors.

She explains, "These nerves are part of a finely webbed

neural relay system which transmits arousal information between the clitoral/corpus cavernosal nerve endings back to the sacral spine (S2–4) and back again." It is this spinal cord reflex that builds arousal. So, she continues, massaging these arousal nerves that "wrap around and dive into the substance of the prostate gland ... amplifies or increases the number of stimuli relaying to the sacral spine," thereby creating the feelings of intense arousal that are associated with prostate massage.

Meanwhile, "our sensory nerves may tell us (internally) how the prostate gland feels about being massaged (level of touch, sensation of vibration, sensation of pain, etc.), but they are not directly related to how we experience the arousal of the pelvic plexus... So in this way, although we aim at the prostate as something to massage for sexual pleasure, it is more the road sign that tells us where the nerves of the pelvic plexus are."

The neurological source of female G-spot sensations has been an active area of research for quite some time. We hope that, as prostate stimulation gains more widespread attention as a source of pleasure for men, research will be directed to this area as well.

THE ROOT CHAKRA

In Tantra, there is a practice of getting in touch with the flow of energy inside your body. With practice, many people can learn to feel a flow of energy inside them and to circulate it in the body. The energy is called *Kundalini*. Practitioners say they can feel it move along certain channels and gather in pools in certain areas the body. The pools, which are mapped vertically through the torso and head, are called *chakras* (pronounced SHOCK-rahs).

What does this have to do with the prostate? The prostate is said to be connected to the *root chakra* in men. The root chakra is located just below the prostate and it is the seat of Kundalini. This is significant because the way to have a full-body orgasm is to draw the Kundalini energy up from the root chakra and circulate it throughout the body.

We spoke with Jan Robinson, a Certified Ipsalu Tantra Kriya Yoga Instructor, about the relationship of the prostate to the root chakra, and she explained that because of the prostate's connection to this chakra, "when [a man's] prostate is stimulated, either directly or indirectly, his root energy gets stimulated too."

She also explained that this usually doesn't happen with traditional intercourse, unless the fellow is involved in Tantric practices: "One of the drawbacks for a man in conventional sexual intercourse is that his root chakra [typically] does *not* get stimulated. This means his Kundalini [...] the energy of evolutionary consciousness, the source of supercharged full-body orgasm, is not awakened."

There are Tantra techniques to activate the root chakra and bring the energy up the body that don't involve prostate massage but rather breathing, meditation, or muscular contractions. But prostate massage is a great way to do it too!

It's also interesting to note that this idea that prostate stimulation can stimulate the root energy, awakening the Kundalini and allowing for full-body orgasms, is quite consistent with what men commonly say about prostate stimulation: that it tends to feel more full-bodied than cock play alone and can feel like waves coursing through the body.

Here is one interesting possible explanation for this: some have suggested that the chakras correspond to the nerve plexuses, such as the pelvic plexus, that run vertically through the torso.

SOURCES OF QUOTES

Michael Thomas Ford, *Ultimate Gay Sex* (DK Publishing, 2004), 23.
Alice Kahn Ladas, Beverly Whipple, and John D. Perry, *The G Spot and Other Discoveries About Human Sexuality* (Holt Paperback, 1982), 134.

4

HYGIENE

Among the men we surveyed about prostate play, fear of "the mess" was the number one concern men of *all* sexual orientations faced when they started out. This anxiety can be a big, distracting turn-off. Nothing will kill an orgasm faster than a little voice in your head shouting "Smelly? Messy? Gross?" and wondering whether your partner will run out the door in disgust.

A certain level of caution is a good thing, since there are some realistic cleanliness concerns, such as diseases that can be contracted through anal play and contact with fecal matter. (We discuss this below.) But the anxiety that some people feel when exploring anal play may have more to do with stigma than with these rational concerns.

It may be difficult to cleanse the reputation of the ass, but thankfully the real thing cleans up quite easily. With soap and warm water, the anus will be clean and fresh smelling, just like any other part of your body. There may be a faint residual odor—this is a natural odor and usually not an offensive one. In fact, as with many body scents, some people really dig it.

If you have concerns about cleanliness, washing before play can help ease your mind considerably, both by cleaning things up and helping you relax. Take a shower or a bath and suds up your hole with a mild soap that does not contain dyes, scents, or harsh chemicals, as these may irritate the anus and cause itching. You can insert your finger a little bit into the hole, but don't go deeper than the anal sphincters because soap can irritate the rectum—the last thing you want before a date! Rinse thoroughly. Washing is particularly advisable if your play includes rimming (oral-anal sex), as there is high risk for catching intestinal parasites or certain STIs if the receiving partner is infected.

It may also help to know that if you have a good diet (lots of fiber, not much grease), there shouldn't be much residue in the rectum. In fact, it should be pretty empty right up until you have that "gotta go to the bathroom" sensation. However, if your stool is loose or if you have constipation, there might be something left behind. Changing your diet can help a lot, but if the diarrhea or constipation are the side effects of a medication, there may not be much you can do.

When you're new to anal play, it might feel like you need to go to the bathroom. Most of the time when this happens, you don't really have to go. It is simply that your body is taking the signal of a full rectum to mean what it usually means—time to stop at the john! So you feel the urge to go, even though in all likelihood no stool is present. It may take a few times before your body learns to reinterpret the sensation and the "gotta go" feeling stops coming. To make that easier, hold still and breathe with deep, slow inhalations and deep, slow exhalations.

QUICK TIPS FOR MORE HYGIENIC ANAL PLAY

- Wear gloves to keep your hands clean.

- Put a towel on the bed to keep the sheets from getting dirty. Keep a hand towel or baby wipes nearby, in case you need to wipe up. And maybe a third towel so you have somewhere to put your used toys when you're done with them.

- If you're concerned about odors, light some incense or a scented candle.

- Use toys that are made from easy-to-clean materials, such as silicone, intramed, or hard plastic. Taking care of these products is simple: wash them well with soap and hot water. You can also put silicone toys in boiling water for five minutes to disinfect them.

- If your favorite toy isn't so easy to clean, or if you're not sure, just cover it with a condom.

- Shower before play and wash the anal opening with a mild soap. Rinse well.

- If you want, you can clear the contents of the rectum beforehand with an enema. Disposable enema bulbs are available from most drugstores. Just be sure to look into enema safety before you give yourself one! (See below for more info.)

- An enema is not the only way to clear out fecal matter. As crude as this may sound, you can check yourself for large chunks by simply reaching in and feeling around. Put on a glove, dab on some lube, insert your finger, and feel around. If you find anything, try to hook your finger around it and sweep it out.

ENEMAS

Some people like to have an enema to rinse out the rectum before penetration. It isn't a necessity; lots of people do without it. As mentioned above, there usually isn't that much poop in there. However, some people like the feeling of inner cleanliness and the peace of mind that an enema brings. Also, feces can be abrasive to the rectal tissue, so an enema may add to your comfort and the longevity of your session. If you are playing with large objects, lots of motion, or for long periods of time, an enema may be a good idea.

Enema Guidelines

Here are some pointers on how to give yourself an enema.

Use the right water

If you don't drink the water that comes out of your tap without filtering it, why would you put it in your rectum? Use the same filtered water that you drink for your enemas. Adding salt to the water makes it easier on your body because saline water won't absorb salt from your body. Add 1/2 teaspoon of uniodized sea salt per 8 ounces of water (1.25 ml of salt for 240 ml of water). It doesn't have to be exact, and a bit less salt is easier on the body than a bit too much. If you're only occasionally doing enemas, salt may not be necessary, but if you do them regularly, it's a good idea.

Water temperature

The water you use for your enema should be warm. Not too hot—that'll burn! And not too cold—that could give you cramps. Test the temperature on your wrist before squirting it up your ass. It should feel warm and pleasant. If it's too hot or too cold for your wrist, chances are it won't feel nice on your insides, either.

Hold it in

Once you take the water in, hold it for a few minutes or as long as you comfortably can. This allows the water to loosen up the solid matter as much as possible so that more of it can be flushed out.

Repeat the rinse

It is common to repeat the rinse—fill the rectum and then empty it two or three times in one enema session, until the water runs clear. Don't do it any more than that, as it may irritate the lining of the tissue (which won't help you out on your hot date later).

Time it!

Usually, if you're doing a shallow rinse, all the water comes out very quickly. If you're doing a deeper rinse, most of it will come out within 15 minutes, usually in a first and second wave. However, if you take in a lot of water, some of it may remain inside, deep in the bowels. This remaining fluid may come insistently to your attention up to an hour later, so leave at least an hour for the enema to clear. Allowing a little time also gives your rectum a chance to settle after the disruption of the enema, which can feel a little uncomfortable when you are new.

Don't overdo it

Every time you have an enema, you are affecting the state of your intestinal microflora. If you are rinsing too many times and too often, you may disrupt the balance, and this can cause disturbances in your bowel function.

Fleet and Bulb Enemas

A Fleet enema (a trade name) or bulb enema consists of a small bottle with a narrowed tip. You fill it with water, insert the tip up your ass, and squeeze the bottle to squirt the water inside you. They can be purchased at most drugstores. The Fleet enema is disposable. It comes in two versions: one with a laxative and one without. Get the laxative-free version, or, if you can only find the laxative version, dump out the solution, rinse the bottle, and fill it with saline water. You can refill it and reuse it a few times in one session, but they're not meant to be used for more than one occasion. They're very handy when you're traveling, though. Bulb enemas can be washed and reused.

Both of these are fairly small bottles, so they give a shallow cleanse. Since the prostate isn't very deep, this may be all you need. To rinse a little deeper, take in the water, hold it inside you, and refill the bottle and give yourself several more fillings before you release all the water at once.

Bag Enemas

A bag enema holds more water, so it can rinse deeper into the GI tract. This thorough cleanse is especially popular for people who are into large objects, fisting, deeper penetration, or long-duration play. Some like it so much that they use it for any kind of anal penetration.

It consists of a rubber or plastic bag that you fill with water and an outlet tube through which the water flows. You insert the lubricated tip of the tube into your ass, then open a valve to let the water flow in. The bag should be higher than the tube so that the water flows naturally with gravity and the air bubbles go to the top of the bag and not into your GI tract. (Air bubbles can give you cramps, just like when you have gas.) However, you don't need to elevate the bag so high that the water comes rushing in forcefully.

Be careful of the mud factor! Introducing any type of enema might make what would have been only a few traces of poop into a mess of sludge. You may have to repeat the enema a second or third time before the water runs clear.

SAFER SEX BARRIERS

If you think that using barriers is a turn-off, you may find that a few hot sessions of prostate massage quickly give new meaning to the sound of a snapping glove! Some people resist barriers because they aren't used to them and think they will be a hassle. While a barrier may be a little awkward at first, with a little practice, you may find it's just the opposite: barriers add convenience to your sex life. They make it easier to switch from one activity to another without having to make a trip to the sink to wash up. If you use gloves to finger your partner's ass, then you can slip them off afterward and you don't have to worry about putting your hand down on a nice clean pillow.

Using gloves, condoms, and dental dams for anal play can help both partners feel more relaxed about keeping things clean. It also makes your play safer by reducing the risk of contracting an infection. There are many ways that infections can be spread during anal play:

- Oral-anal contact (rimming) can transmit intestinal parasites and some STIs (sexually transmitted infections).

- Accidental oral contact with shit (from unwashed hands) can transmit parasites and may transmit some STIs.

- Unprotected anal sex can transmit STIs, especially for the receiver.

- Unprotected anal intercourse puts the giver at risk for prostatitis, since bacteria can enter the urethra and travel up to the prostate. (See chapter 14, Prostate Health.)

- Sharing toys may carry risk for STI transmission.

Gloves

In addition to keeping the hands clean, gloves can also nicely smooth over any rough areas on your hands so that the receiver gets a smoother ride. Of course, gloves that are poorly fitted and bunchy won't feel much better! Often the receiver can feel it when the gloves are wrinkled, especially at the anal opening, where wrinkles tend to gather. Pull them on snugly so the fingers are as smooth and wrinkle-free as possible.

If wrinkles gather at the base of the finger, use plenty of lube on that area. You might even favor motions that minimize the friction at the anus, such as curling the fingers and keeping the hand stationary rather than moving fingers in and out. Different brands and materials of gloves fit a little differently, so shop around. A snugger fit means less friction for the receiver.

To reduce the obtrusiveness of wearing a glove, try this trick: put the glove on, squirt a little lube into the glove, and work it down to the fingertips. The feeling of wetness on the inside almost makes it feel like you aren't wearing a glove at all. It also reduces the bunching effect that can happen with gloves that don't fit quite right.

Gloves come in a variety of materials. Latex gloves are inexpensive and easy to find at a drugstore. This material is thin and flexible, and many prefer the texture, since it has so much give. Make sure you don't use them with any oil-based lubricant, such as Vaseline, baby oil, or massage oil. Oil breaks down latex, and this may cause the barrier to break. Unfortunately, many people have latex sensitivities and can't use latex barriers; there are vinyl and nitrile options for them. You can get gloves in these materials at some drugstores. You can also purchase them online from dental and medical suppliers, and from many sex toy retailers. If the plain white glove feels too medical to you, find a color that feels a bit more "oh-la-la!" A wide variety of colors are available, including black. You can find them online. Just don't get the loose vinyl gloves that are used in food service, since they get really bunched up.

If you choose not to wear gloves for anal penetration, be sure to wash your hands thoroughly with soap and warm water, including under the fingernails. Also, bear in mind that some odor may linger on your skin even after you've washed.

Condoms

Condoms—not just for penises anymore! They're also a great way to keep toys clean, especially if you're planning to share them. Condoms are a particularly good idea for toys that are porous. Porous materials like jelly rubber and softskin cannot be sanitized due to microscopic holes that can hold on to whatever they come into contact with.

Some people find that they have latex sensitivities which can cause irritation or a burning feeling. Fortunately, there are other options these days, including polyisoprene and polyurethane condoms. If you can't find them at your drugstore, check some of the sex-positive sex toy companies online. They usually have a good range of products. Using condoms isn't difficult, but there are some things you can do to make them more effective, whether you're using them on a toy or on a penis.

- Latex and polyisoprene condoms should be stored away from heat because exposure to higher temperatures makes these materials brittle and more likely to break. It's fine to stick one in your pocket when you're going on a date, but don't carry it in your wallet or keep it in a drawer near a heater.

- All condoms sold in the US have a five-year expiration date and it's printed on every wrapper. If you discover some condoms in the back of your drawer, be sure to check the date and make sure they're still good.

- Open the wrapper at the corner instead of tearing it in the middle. It's possible to tear the condom accidentally.

- If you're putting the condom on a penis, apply a little lubricant to the inside of the condom before rolling it on. Just a dab in the unrolled condom keeps the lube at the head of the penis, where it is more sensitive, and off the shaft, so it doesn't make the condom slide off.

- If you're putting the condom on a toy, roll it all the way down and, if possible, over the base. This will give you maximum coverage.

- Never use oils or lubricants containing oils with latex or polyisoprene condoms. Oils make them break. If you want to see it for yourself, blow up a condom like a balloon and tie it off. Apply a few drops of oil—massage oil, olive oil, baby oil, or any other you have handy. Rub it in with your hand and the condom will pop within a minute. (Polyurethane condoms are safe to use with oils, but they're not as sheer or as stretchy as latex or polyisoprene condoms.)

- Be sure to use plenty of lube on the outside of the condom. Since condoms have a bit more friction than other materials, you'll need a little extra help to keep things slippery.

- If the condom is on a penis, check every so often

to make sure it's still there during sex, since they can slip off, especially if the penis gets a bit soft. This is not usually a problem with a toy, since toys don't get soft while you use them. That's one of the advantages of them! And after ejaculation, hold the base of the condom to keep from leaving it behind as the penis softens.

- Throw the used condom out in the trash. Flushing it can lead to clogged pipes.

Another option that works well for prostate play is the FC2, also known as the female condom. It's a loose pouch of nitrile meant to be inserted into the vagina instead of rolled onto the penis, but it works just fine for anal play too. For anal use, first take out the removable inner ring. This ring is meant to hold the FC2 against the cervix, but it's not necessary for anal play. Be careful to insert the finger, toy, or penis into the condom rather than between the condom and the skin.

Dental Dams

Dental dams are thin sheets of latex or nitrile that are used in some dental procedures. They were brought into our bedrooms as a form of protection for cunnilingus and anal-ingus (rimming).

If you want to use a dental dam, here are a few tips. Put lube on the side of the dam that will go on your partner. Then lay the dam out over the area to be licked. The lube will not only feel nice and give your partner a sense of wetness to the touch, but will also help keep the dam clinging to the skin, which will make it easier to keep it in place.

Dental dams are available at lots of sex-positive toy shops. You can also make a dental dam from a flavored condom by unrolling it, snipping off the tip, and then cutting down the side to form a rectangle. Another option is to use plastic wrap, which comes in many colors and can cover a larger area. Contrary to popular belief, microwavable plastic wrap works just fine—the small pores don't open until steam heats them up.

HAIR REMOVAL

Many people of all genders enjoy the appearance of a thick, dark forest on their partner's genitals. But there are many benefits to grooming your anus. Some men have especially hairy assholes—the hair can get in the way and lead to pulling during penetration. Also, the hair tends to absorb the lube that you are trying get into the hole, which means less gets where you want it to go.

To clear the path, some men choose to shave or wax their assholes. When the hole is hairless, it's easier to get the area nice and clean—both before and after play. It also allows the whole surface of asshole and perineum to be evenly stroked. And some really like the look of a smooth bottom! As an aside, lots of men are also shaving around their cock these days. Many men find that it makes their cock look bigger, which is nice for the size queens.

If you don't want the full shave or wax, you can simply

trim the hair to make it more manageable. This is a nice way to sidestep the five o'clock shadow on your tender parts. You can use an electric hair trimmer or some blunt-tipped scissors to give yourself a trim around the hole.

If your ass cheeks are hairy, you might just shave the hole and the crack, rather than shaving both cheeks and ending up looking like you are wearing a pair of furry chaps. Or, you could shave the crack and use a hair removal cream on the cheeks. Don't use these products on the hole! They can burn and irritate the skin, which is the last thing you want before playtime!

Shaving

If you choose to shave, start by trimming as described above. The shorter the hair, the easier it is to get a close shave. Make sure you have a good, sharp razor—avoid the cheap disposable kind. If you wouldn't use it on your face, don't use it on the sensitive skin of your asshole. A dull razor won't cut as effectively, which means more irritation. Red bumps and ingrown hairs are uncomfortable and none too pretty. Replace the razor regularly to make sure it is sharp.

Itching is quite common when the hair starts to grow back. This is because the hair was cut so close that it is below the surface of the skin, and it causes itchiness as it finds its way back out. To minimize the itching, and to avoid ingrown hairs, gently scrub the shaved area with a hard sponge and warm soapy water before you shave, and daily for 2–3 days afterward. This removes dead skin cells that may be blocking the hair follicles. If you shave regularly, the itching usually stops.

When choosing a shaving cream, chances are you won't find a product marketed to men for shaving pubic hair. You can try a product that is made for shaving the face—especially if it is made for sensitive skin. (The skin of the anus is very sensitive and prone to irritation.) If you apply a cream or gel and it stings, rinse it off right away and don't use it again. Likewise, if you are shaving your ass regularly and you find that your anus is irritated, itchy, or red, discontinue the product and see if these symptoms clear up.

Some men use hair conditioner or unscented lotion—this not only lubricates the razor as it glides over the skin but also hydrates the hair, making it softer and easier to cut. To maximize this effect, leave the lotion on for a minute before you shave.

When you are ready to begin, lay a mirror on the floor and squat over it so you have a clear view of what you are doing. Trim the hair if you haven't done so already. Before you apply the shaving product, note the direction of the hair growth: as with your face, you want to shave with the direction of the hair, not against it. Reaching between your legs, gently hold the skin taught with your free hand while you shave with the other. Go slowly and feel your way. Use short strokes and rinse the razor frequently to remove buildup from the cutting surface.

Resist the temptation to press hard or run the razor repeatedly over the same spot. You may not be able to get a perfect shave on the first try, but if you keep running the razor over the same spot it will probably get irritated. It is better to repeat the shave in a day or two than to go too far and get razor burn. And on that subject, if you want to be smooth-shaven for a special night and you've never shaved before, do two shaves: once a few days before and again on the night of the date.

Waxing

Some people prefer to wax because the skin stays smooth longer: usually 3–6 weeks. When the hair does grow back, the tips are soft, since it's new fresh hair rather than sharp pointy tips of cut hair. Of course, waxing has its downside. (*Rip!*—Ouch!) And the angles required means that it will be very difficult to wax yourself down there.

We recommend getting it done professionally. There are many waxing salons that serve both men and women. Call the salon in advance to ask if they offer the "male Brazilian" wax. Make sure that you see someone who is licensed and who has experience working with men. The price range is generally $25–$50.

Often a Brazilian wax includes some or all of the pubic hair, the shaft, the scrotum, and the perineum, according to your preference. It is likely to hurt more the first time and to be less painful on subsequent visits as your skin gets used to it. It will hurt less if you take a pain killer one hour before the procedure.

Alternatively, you could do it at home if you have a willing friend or lover you feel comfortable asking. Home wax kits are available at most drugstores and are very affordable. However, if you are going the DIY route, do not wax your balls! The skin of the scrotum is thin and loose and doesn't generally take well to waxing. Sometimes the wax can take off a layer of skin. Most professionals, if they do wax the scrotum, use a special wax on this area because the usual product does not work. If you want a smooth scrotum and you are going DIY, wax the rest and then shave the balls.

After waxing, expect the skin to be tender for the rest of the day following the wax, and don't plan to have any sexual activity during that time. If you've been cringing while reading this, note that while much of the hair removal may hurt, when you wax right around the asshole it actually feels rather good. Surprised? Try it. You may see what we mean.

5

PENETRATION 101

THE PROSTATE AND THEN SOME

For a lot of men, the prostate is a major part of what makes receiving anal penetration feel good. For many, it is the main event, and for some it is the only reason why they go up there in the first place. But the prostate is not the only thing that makes anal penetration feel good for a man. Although in this book we focus more on the prostate and less on anal pleasure generally, we'd like to take a minute here to tell you about some reasons why going in the back door can be fun.

The anus (the puckered anal opening) has a very high concentration of nerve endings, which means that touching this area can generate a lot of sensation. Many people enjoy a variety of different kinds of touch, from very light caresses to medium pressure. The nerves that supply the anus happen to be branches of the same nerve that supplies the cock and balls, so it's no surprise that anal stimulation can feel so good.

Once you get past the anus and into the rectum (the tube that makes up the final 6–8 inches of your digestive tract), there are fewer nerve endings, so it is less sensitive to caresses but still sensitive to pressure. A lot of people really like the sensation of being filled up and having pressure applied to the rectal walls on all sides. This is one reason why using a butt plug or being fucked with an in-and-out motion can feel good.

Even though prostate pleasure may be the focus for a lot of guys, we've heard from men who have had their prostate removed for the treatment of prostate cancer and still love to have their bottoms poked. They report that their sensation is reduced, unfortunately, but that it is still pleasurable. This points to the fact that the prostate is not the only source of pleasure in that area: the nerves of the anus and rectum also make their contributions.

FROM OUR SURVEY:
"NOT ALL ANAL PENETRATION IS FOCUSED ON STIMULATING THE PROSTATE.
HOW OFTEN IS P-SPOT PLEASURE A CENTRAL PART OF YOUR ANAL PLAY?"

"Not often."

"All of it."

"Most anal play includes prostate play."

"More of a warm-up to other things. Strap-on and such. But in all anal penetration you will rub the P-spot some during the act."

"More on the foreplay portion of my play. But it is clearly part of all anal play."

"Some of my anal play is external and focuses on stimulating the erectile tissue around the opening. Whenever anal play includes penetration, P-spot pleasure is very central."

"When engaging in anal play, I always make some attempt to stimulate the prostate, and then see how the person responds. Sometimes they enjoy it, other times it seems to be too much sensation for them or they have no significant response, so I move on to other activities."

"I don't know if I've reached my P-spot or not. Either way it feels great."

"A quarter of the time it is the focus, but it usually is stroked right before and during orgasm."

"It hasn't really been a focal point of the anal play I do; mostly, if I've stimulated the prostate at all, I've done it by accident."

"Always important, not usually the sole focus."

"Always. In fact if it doesn't involve prostate play then it's not inter-esting/fun/pleasurable to me."

"About half of the time."

"It's the only anal play."

"Always...as a way to open up the asshole for further fucking...and just on it's own...finding the sweet spot with my fingers."

Getting Started

When you are first starting off with anal play, your body is learning two new things: how to physically relax the anal muscles, and how to receive this stimulation as pleasurable. Like anything else that's unfamiliar, you might not get it right away. Your first few anal experiences may feel unremarkable. In fact, it is common for there to be some discomfort the first few times.

Being turned on usually makes anal play a lot easier and more fun. The more turned on you are, the more your brain is likely to interpret new sensations as enjoyable. In fact, you might try starting your exploration of anal penetration by including or even focusing on some other kind of stimulation, such as masturbation or oral sex. Some people eventually find anal play (internal and external, with or without intentional prostate stimulation) to be a pleasure all by itself. Others prefer it as an add-on to their favorite way to play. Either way, as long as it's feeling good, go for it!

An entire book can be written on anal penetration—in fact, there are quite a few. So here we only cover the basics. See the Resources for a list of how-to books and DVDs about anal play.

You Need a Map!

If you're going to go looking for the prostate, you need a map of the surrounding territory.

First things first: the anus. This is the puckered, pink circle that forms the anal opening. Under the skin are the anal sphincters: two rings of muscle that separate the rectum from the outside world. You can think of them as two donuts, one on top of the other. When you slip your finger inside, you are sliding it through the donut holes.

The "upper" donut (the one closer to your head) is called the internal anal sphincter. It is continuous with the involuntary smooth muscle of the intestines. The "lower" donut, the external anal sphincter, sits underneath the internal sphincter, but it also comes up and around it and connects to other muscles of the pelvis. The external anal sphincter is a part of the PC group, the group of muscles that convulse rhythmically during orgasm.

The ring formed by the sphincters opens up when they are relaxed and closes in when they are flexed. Since the sphincters are each made of a different kind of muscle, they work a little differently when they relax and tighten. The external sphincter (that's the lower donut in the stack—the one closest to the outside of your body) is made of skeletal muscle. That means that it can be flexed and relaxed voluntarily, like your hand or your foot. The internal sphincter (the top donut) is an entirely different matter. Since the internal sphincter is continuous with the smooth muscle of the digestive tract, it is controlled by a subdivision of the nervous system that is not under voluntary control, just like the rest of the intestines. This can sometimes make it difficult to deliberately relax it.

If you are in a truly relaxed state and you allow the external sphincter to open, the internal one often follows suit. But you can't fake it, because your involuntary nervous system knows whether or not your interest in being penetrated is sincere. If you are nervous or anxious, the sphincters tend to tighten up—your body doesn't care if the reason you're stressed is because you were stuck in traffic, you had a busy day, or you're nervous about anal penetration hurting. Fortunately, with a little practice, it usually becomes easier to encourage the internal sphincter to open up.

Once you get past the anal muscles, you're in the rectum. You'll notice it's much roomier here. The rectum is an expandable tube with thin, soft walls and gentle folds, and it's lined with a mucous membrane to protect the delicate tissue. Because of the lining, it feels moist to the touch, though there isn't usually enough moisture to allow comfortable penetration without lube.

It is important to know that the rectum is not straight. Quick exercise: grab a piece of scrap paper and draw an S. Make it a very tall, thin S so that the curves are soft, as if the S is being squeezed in a vise from left to right. Now hold the paper up to your right side. You are now a cutaway diagram of the rectum! Viewed from the side, this is roughly the way the rectum curves: from the anus it moves first toward the belly, then toward the back, and finally toward the belly again.

Why is this important? Because, as Jack Morin points out in *Anal Pleasure and Health*, if you are aiming too far toward the front of the body as you go in deeper, you may run right into the first curve. Poke!—ouch. This is especially relevant to prostate play, since when you are looking for the prostate you are aiming toward the front wall of the rectum.

This tends to be less of an issue with fingers, which are shorter and can easily feel where they are going. With a cock, a dildo, or other toys of significant length, it is much easier to bump painfully into the first curve, especially if you are doing short strokes right over the prostate and then suddenly plunge deeper. To avoid this, go slow when you are moving deeper and adjust the angle so that you are not pointing too sharply to the front of the body.

PENETRATION: THE BASICS

Whether you're on your own or with a partner, here are some useful guidelines for painless and pleasurable anal penetration.

Start Solo

If you are new to receiving anal penetration, we recommend that you fly solo for your first few tries. Even if your partner is quite experienced and skilled, doing it by yourself allows you to get comfortable with the new sensation in a pressure-free environment. You can focus entirely on yourself without distraction or performance anxiety. This should also alleviate concerns about "the mess."

It can be really helpful to play with your own ass before you play with someone else's! Everyone has an asshole—men, women, cisgender, transgender, genderqueer—we've all got 'em! So no matter who you are or what your orientation, you can play with your own bottom and it'll make you better equipped to pleasure someone else's, since you will know how it feels (ahem) firsthand.

Trim Your Nails!

You'll also want to make sure that your fingernails are short and smooth. Run them along your lips to check for any rough edges and file them down as needed. Gloves can also cover up any rough spots. If you have long nails that you want to keep, tear some cotton balls into thirds or quarters and stuff them into the fingers of a glove with a pencil. When you put the glove on, push the cotton under the tips of your nails. You won't get as much sensation, but you'll protect both your partner and your manicure.

The Importance of Being Lubricated

The rectum does not self-lubricate, and without lube, anal penetration can be uncomfortable, painful, or even injurious. With lube, it will feel slick and smooth, plus it's a lot safer for the delicate tissues of the rectum. Even if you think there's enough, put a little more on your fingers and apply it to the anus and rectum.

One of the functions of the rectum is to absorb water from your waste and back into your body, so if you're using a water-based lubricant, it will dry out after a while. Tell your partner when things are getting sticky, so you can apply more lubricant. With some brands your partner can add a splash of water to rejuvenate the dried-out lube. There are a lot of different kinds of lubricants these days, so we've written much more about them and how to pick one. See chapter 11, Toys, for more information.

If It Hurts, Don't Do It!

If you experience any pain, stop what you're doing and don't force it. You could hurt yourself. If your body isn't ready for more, listen to it. Even if you're experienced with anal play, your body sometimes might not be into it.

Some men ask about desensitizing sprays or creams. Others may use drugs or alcohol to dull the pain. We do not recommend this. While we don't think it's a problem to have a drink or two, if you're not in a state of mind where you can pay attention to how things feel or tell your partner what's going on, it's probably a good idea to hold off on prostate fun for another time. Pain is an important warning sign of potential damage, and if you can't feel pain, you are at risk of hurting yourself without realizing it.

Rather than trying to cover up or push through the pain, it's actually much more effective and a lot more pleasurable to learn how to relax the pelvic floor. After all, if you're turning off the nerve endings so you can't feel pain, you are also turning off those same nerve endings to the good sensations, which are the whole point in the first place! Is it any fun to kiss someone after getting a shot of Novocain at the dentist?

Some sex educators seem to suggest that anyone can have pleasurable anal penetration, but in our opinion, that's simply not true. For example, sometimes a previous injury or trauma makes penetration uncomfortable or painful. If that's your experience, perhaps the best way to keep anal play from hurting is not to do it. There are plenty of other fun ways to enjoy sex.

On the other hand, quite a few people who have had unfortunate experiences that made anal penetration painful have discovered that by going slowly and carefully they can turn that around. Whatever your situation, if it hurts, something needs to change. There are a lot of things you can do to ease pain if it arises.

IF IT HURTS

- Slow down or stop the motion. If you're not already on your back, lie down, relax, and take several deep breaths, then see if the sensation passes. If your partner is controlling the motion, make sure to establish in advance whether "stop" means "hold still" or "pull out."

- Introduce something pleasurable, like stroking your cock. Adding familiar pleasures to the experience makes it easier for your body to decide that anal play feels good. This, in turn, may spark a stronger desire to be penetrated, and that can help the muscles of the pelvic floor release.

- Apply more lube to reduce friction.

- If you've inserted an object, remove it and give your ass a break. Be sure to remove it slowly and exhale as you withdraw: even if it hurts, going too quickly can make it hurt more.

- If the object is too big, scale back to a smaller object.

- If none of this helps, call it a day and move on to some other kind of stimulation. Sometimes anal play just doesn't work, but that doesn't mean you can't do it again another day.

SLOW AND STEADY WINS THE RACE

"Ironically, going slowly gets you in faster."

—CHARLES SILVERSTEIN AND FELICE PICANO

Remember the lesson of the tortoise and the hare: slow and steady wins the race! It is important to pace yourself as you explore anal penetration. Negative experiences can set you back further than if you had taken your time in the first place. Rushing can lead to discomfort or pain, which can turn your body off to the sensations and make it less likely that you will feel pleasure: "In general, subjecting any area to pain will cause a tightening, an internal withdrawal of feeling from that area. This will result in a numbness and desensitization of that area."[12]

For your first few times, don't go too far too fast, even if it feels good—you may have a sore bottom tomorrow.

"Sometimes anal play just hurts, and that kills the prostate pleasure."

Don't dive in the deep end with rapid motion or very large objects. Sex educator Tristan Taormino suggests two fingers for first-time anal penetration, and we think this is reasonable. Of course, it depends on the size of the fingers—

one might be plenty enough, and that's perfectly fine.

Some people believe that anal penetration is always painful and that the only way to get to the pleasure is to push through the pain. This is not true! Many, many people regularly experience anal penetration that feels good the whole time and doesn't hurt.

If you stop what you are doing and let the pain subside, you may be able to find the pleasure you are seeking. In most cases, pushing through the pain only makes it hurt more. And taking the pain today will make it even harder to have pain-free penetration next time. Your ass will remember.

In his book *Anal Pleasure and Health,* Jack Morin explains how memories are stored in the body. Painful memories translate into muscular tension, so the only way to relieve the tension is to slowly replace the bad memories with good ones. You can't do it by creating more bad ones.[13]

We interviewed a man about his experience receiving penetration. We asked, "Was it ever painful for you?" and he said, "Sometimes, yeah. But I also have a high pain tolerance and don't mind pain." Interestingly,

"I used to believe that there would be the pain at first and then it would slowly become more pleasurable after that, but I've since realized that if you gradually work your way into it, it's fun times the whole way."

he was someone who had never found pleasure in anal penetration and had turned away from it. The point is: maybe you can take the pain, but we'd be willing to bet that it won't do you much good. Once it starts hurting, it is unlikely that the pain will give way to pleasure if you push through it.

Relax the Mind

Anal play definitely works best when you're in a relaxed state of mind because our emotions affect our physical states. If you have a mental block such as a nagging anxiety repeating in your head, or if you're stressed out from a busy day, it can trigger muscular tension.

Do you ever grit your teeth when you're stressed? Well, the jaw is not the only place where people tighten when feeling anxiety. Many people also squeeze their pelvic muscles, including the anal sphincters. This is why someone who is uptight may be called "anal-retentive" or a "tight-ass." Men especially are prone to keeping their pelvic muscles and anal sphincters overly tight. If your sphincters are clamped shut, it will be more difficult to get in there.

To help yourself relax mentally, eliminate distractions as much as possible. If you have nagging thoughts that are pulling you away from the experience at hand, put them to rest by addressing them. Worried someone is going to come in? Lock the door. Afraid the roommates will hear you and they'll *know* what you're doing? Put on some music.

It may help ease your mind to take a bath or meditate. Put aside enough time so you aren't rushed, and make sure you have everything you need before you start. You might gather lube, a drip towel, gloves, something to wipe your hands with, toys, and a towel to lay on the floor for your discard pile.

Above all, take it easy. Try not to try too hard. We've spoken with men who treated anal penetration and the search for the prostate like a desperate climb for a fabled treasure at the top of a mountain. They would try and try, and then wonder why it continued to elude them. With so much mental energy and effort, no wonder they weren't enjoying themselves!

If this is you, you may benefit from an attitude adjustment. Instead of trying to make your play conform to your expectations, release the impulse to control and let each moment be what it is. As is often the case with sex, sometimes it's easier to get what we want when we let go of reaching for it.

Breathe Deep to Help You Relax

The way you breathe can literally change your state of mind and body. Taking short, shallow breaths is what we do in "go" mode, the activation state of the body, so breathing that way tends to put you in an active head space. Deep, long, easy breaths tend to put you in a state of relaxation. Intentionally regulating your breathing by softening it and relaxing it actually makes you feel more relaxed. And that makes it easier to let the sphincters open to allow penetration.

Breathe deeply and slowly to relax. Make sure you do a complete inhale *and* a complete exhale. Many men, told to breathe deep, take a deep breath in and hold it. Holding your breath takes effort! We're going for less effort and more ease.

It's not just about taking in a lot of air on the inhale—it's about releasing it on the exhale. The exhale is the more relaxing part of the breath. In fact, if you pay attention, you may be able to notice your anus tightening a bit when you breathe in and relaxing as you breathe out.

There's also a common tendency, when told to exhale, to push the air out forcefully. Again, that's effort. What you want is less effort, more release of effort. Try letting it out softly and smoothly, as if of its own will, rather than pushing it out forcibly.

Many people find that the initial penetration works best when they exhale at the same time. Take a slow, deep breath and then slowly let it out as the finger or toy enters your anus. If you're doing it with a partner, breathing together can be a great way to sync up, feel connected, and ensure that the giver is paying attention to the receiver.

Relax the Body

To allow something inside your ass, your sphincter muscles need to relax in order to open up. A lot of people believe (mistakenly) that when you enter the ass, you gain access by stretching the sphincters like a rubber band. This may be the origin of the myth that anal sex will put you in adult diapers: that by stretching them over and over, they will become over-stretched and, also like a rubber band, lose their elasticity and their ability to bounce back to the original state of tension. In fact, plenty of people have been playing with their asses for years without losing sphincter tone or control.

Of course, the sphincter muscles do stretch, like any other muscle, and they may receive some stretch during anal pene-tration, particularly if they tend to be tight. Just like other muscles, the anus is capable of increasing its flexibility over time. This is why people who have lots of anal experience can accommodate larger objects. But, as with those other muscles, you can strain it if you try to stretch it more quickly than it can handle. One sex educator we know compared this to learning to do a split in gymnastics: you wouldn't expect to do it all in one day. Rather, you'd practice regularly and each time you'd be able to go a little lower to the ground. It's the same with penetration. You may not be able to take larger objects right away, but you might eventually, if you increase your flexibility gradually over time.

Relaxing the sphincters is harder than it may sound. We are used to thinking that we have complete control over the actions of our muscles. If you want to flex your hand to make a fist, you do it, and if you want to relax it, you do it, and it's easy. But most people have had a lot more practice flexing and relaxing their hands than their anal sphincters. Chances are, the sphincters are accustomed to releasing only when necessary for a bowel movement. Otherwise, they are held closed by their muscular tone, and perhaps even locked down if you have over-tight muscles. So, it may take some practice to learn how to relax them.

Then again, relaxing the sphincters may come easily to you, especially if you have good muscular awareness. We met a fellow who had only done anal play two or three times before, and he was able to take three fingers like a sip of lemonade because he had done lots of yoga and was very well in touch with his muscles. But for many of us it will not come so easily.

You might find that your brain says to your ass: "please open," and your ass completely ignores this message. It may take a while for you to learn how to convey that relaxation message thoroughly to your ass. A lot of people get in a bind here because they want to relax so they try, try, try. And, ironically, the harder you try, the less likely it is to happen, because trying hard is the opposite of relaxing. Instead, try letting go of the ambition.

Massaging the Sphincters

A good way to get any muscle to relax is to massage it. This applies in a most pleasurable fashion to the sphincters. Before penetration, rub the sphincters softly with lube. You can trace a fingertip in a circle along the ring, or rub up and down over it. Try adding pressure or touching more lightly. You can press-and-release over the whole surface, or rest your finger gently in the middle of the opening, without pushing in.

This kind of attention not only helps the muscles relax, but also feels amazing. The teasing, lingering touch on the outside makes the ass crave penetration and also helps you relax mentally because it feels much less threatening to the hole than a clambering rush for entry. It reassures the ass that you are going slow and taking your time. Soon, the ass is not only relaxed enough for penetration, but begging for it!

It is easy to blast past this phase in your eagerness to plunge deeper and get to the prostate already. However, you do yourself a disservice if you skip this step, because it can be extremely pleasurable and can make what comes later even more enjoyable.

Learning to Relax the Sphincters

As with all new skills, learning to relax the sphincters comes more easily with practice. Most people find that the more often they practice, the easier and faster they can open up. Conversely, if you go for a while without doing anal play, it can take some time to build up the ability again. So expect to take your time if you haven't done it in a while.

Practicing Kegel exercises also helps you gain control over the sphincters. (See chapter 6, Searching for the "Magic Button.") This may seem counterintuitive. The purpose here is not necessarily to strengthen the pelvic muscles; it is to get them toned. When they are toned they are both strong and supple, and they can relax just as easily as they can tense. Getting your PC muscles in shape helps you get in tune with the sphincters and gives you better awareness of them, which will make it easier to relax them.

Try inserting your finger (with lube, please) just a little way into the sphincters and squeeze them so they tighten around your finger. Then give just as much of your attention to relaxing them. Repeat several times, making sure to spend as much time on the release as on the tightening.

MAKING IT FEEL GOOD

You can't just shove something up there and expect it to feel good. (Though if you've been doing this for a while, maybe you can!) When you are trying to get into something new, it helps a lot if you are aroused before you begin. The more turned on you are, the easier penetration can be and the better it'll feel.

Include familiar pleasures. Play with the cock, balls, perineum, thighs, nipples, or whatever else gets the fire burning. Allow your thoughts and fantasies to wander where they will without judging them.

Focus on the ass, stroking it at a slow, leisurely pace. Give the cheeks some attention. You can rub them and squeeze them and gently pull them apart. If you are playing with someone else's ass, jiggle the hips from side to side with your hands, like a massage therapist, to help the muscles of the pelvis relax.

When it's time for penetration, don't just shove in—give the outside some love. Remember what we said about sphincter massage? Use your finger or toy or cock to lavish affection on the hole before entering. Some people like to use their mouths for this—this is called rimming.

When you are ready to slip inside, go very slowly and gently. The sphincters should relax open to allow penetration. You can apply some pressure, but you shouldn't force your way in. Once inside, don't jump straight into movement. Let the ass adjust to being penetrated by holding still for a spell.

You may wish to keep cock play going at the same time. This is a great way to make anal penetration feel good when you are still learning to eroticize it. However, rubbing the cock can make the PC muscles—including the anal sphincters—tighten as a result of the excitement, which makes initial entry difficult, so you may want to let go of the cock for at least a few minutes at the moment of penetration.

Penetration Techniques

There are a few different techniques for getting an object inside you.

- Bear down: With the penetrating object at the opening of your anus, bear down while exhaling, as if having a bowel movement. This opens the sphincters, and you can then slowly let it in.

- Bear down, pull up: Same technique, except this is for those with good PC muscle control. Bear down to let the object in a little, then pull up and in with your PC muscles, so that you are sucking the object into you. Repeat until it's in past the sphincters.

- Press down, slip in: With your fingertip at the hole, push down on the sphincter to hold it slightly open. Imagine the anus as the face of a clock, and press gently at six o'clock to stretch it just a little bit. Release the pressure as you slip in.

Other Tips

If you're using a finger, you'll be able to feel both sphincters. One might be tighter than the other, so go at the pace of the one that's slower to open up. It's more likely to catch up that way than if you try to get it to do more than it wants. Help the sphincters release by *gently* pressing up, down, right, left, to stretch them and encourage them to open.

If you're moving the toy or finger in and out, pay attention to how the sphincters contract and release. When they contract, slow down or hold still. Stroke the cock, massage the perineum, or do something else that feels good. When they release again, you can return to the motion.

Sometimes, even once you get going, it's nice to slow down or even hold still for a few moments. There's an idea in our pleasure culture that more stimulation means more pleasure, but that's not always so. After all, a lot of people enjoy butt plugs because they create a feeling of fullness or pressure without an in-and-out motion. More movement isn't always better.

You might find that one part of the anus feels especially tight or sensitive. Since there are a lot of pelvic muscles, tension in any of them can make relaxing the anus difficult. Gently but firmly press on the area that feels tight and hold the pressure for about 60 seconds. This often helps release the tension more easily than with a more vigorous massage.

Always start with smaller objects and work your way up to larger ones. Fingers are convenient because they come in so many different sizes! You can start with the smallest finger and increase in size. Anytime you change to a wider finger or toy, or add a finger, apply some lube and exhale as you slide it inside, then hold still for a moment to let the ass get used to the new object.

SOURCE OF QUOTE

Charles Silverstein and Felice Picano, *The Joy of Gay Sex*, 3rd ed., fully revised and expanded (HarperCollins, 2003), 92.

CHAPTER

6

SEARCHING FOR
THE "MAGIC BUTTON"

So you want to find the prostate? Great! This is the place to start. We have lots of tips to help you find the prostate and have a good time doing it. Although this chapter focuses on guys who are looking for their own prostate, most of the information will also be useful to those of you who want to find a partner's.

FINDING IT IS NOT JUST ABOUT LOCATION

Before we describe the location of the prostate and how to reach it with your eager fingertips, we have an important point to make: unlike real estate, when it comes to the prostate, it's not just about location. There's more to prostate pleasure than just physically locating the gland.

People often talk about finding the prostate as if that's all you have to do: just push the "magic button" and presto! Instant pleasure! As a result, it is common for a man looking for his prostate to poke and prod all over the front wall of the rectum, and when he's not overcome by waves of ecstasy, he assumes that he simply isn't touching the right area.

We interviewed a guy who had looked for his prostate on multiple occasions with no luck. He had tried with fingers and toys, by himself and with his wife, yet he hadn't felt anything remarkable. He said: "You can read all you want about it, but unless someone [...] knows exactly where to go, you won't find it. With all the experimentation we've done to locate it, I still don't know if we're locating it." This is a common experience and a frustrating one.

It's true that in order to feel prostate sensations, you need to be stimulating the right spot. If you are not contacting the gland because you are too deep, too shallow, or off to one side, then you are not likely to feel much of anything. However, it is also possible to push *exactly on the prostate* and not feel any pleasure at all. One man's partner gave us this account: "I could clearly identify the outline of the prostate, so I was sure that I was in the right place—I've done a lot of this and I know what to look for. But he didn't feel any pleasure. All he felt was 'pressure.'" In other cases, men have reported feeling discomfort, numbness, pain, or an urge to pee when their prostate is massaged.

If you don't feel much right away when your prostate is touched, that doesn't necessarily mean that you haven't found the right spot. The prostate is not a "magic button" that delivers pleasure automatically as soon as you touch it. Many other factors come into play, such as your state of mind and level of arousal. We discuss these factors here.

THE MIND–BODY CONNECTION

People tend to speak of the mind and the body as separate, but in reality, this is just a manner of speaking. The mind and the body are one, and your mental/emotional state can have very real effects on your physical state. A good example of this is people who are afraid of flying, who, because they are feeling fear, unconsciously grip the armrests, giving rise to the expression "white-knuckle flyer." Or people who are thinking about something upsetting may suddenly notice that they are clenching their fists or gritting their teeth. What we call "the mind" and what we call "the body" are interconnected, and our mental states impact what we experience physically.

This applies to sex too. Though some people think of sex as a purely physical affair, your state of mind is just as important for sex as it would be for work or any other activity. Some mental states are ideal for maximizing pleasure and others can actually get in the way of it.

An example of this which many men experience at some point in their lives is the vicious circle of performance anxiety. Let's say that you're sleeping with a new partner for the first time and you are worried about being able to "perform" by getting and keeping an erection. When you feel anxious, your body starts to produce adrenaline, which causes the blood vessels in the penis to constrict. This prevents them from relaxing enough to let in blood to produce an erection. As a result, the anxiety lessens your ability to "perform," ironically causing the very thing that you are worried about.

Another physical effect of strong negative emotions that comes up for sex play is the tightening of the muscles that form the pelvic floor. You've probably seen a scared dog with its tail tucked under its body and its rear end lower to the ground in a fearful posture. People do the same thing: in situations of fear, stress, and pain, the muscles of the pelvic floor can tighten, pulling the tailbone slightly inward between the legs. These muscles are the same ones that you need to relax in order to receive anal penetration, which means yet another vicious circle. If you're worried that penetration may hurt, you might end up with tight pelvic muscles, which makes it less likely that penetration will feel good.

These are very specific, dramatic examples of the mind–body connection, but it can be more subtle too. If you just aren't really in the mood, or you're feeling a little insecure because of something your partner said, or having any other difficult emotions, it may hold you back in the sack. As far as the body's reactions go, it doesn't matter where the negative emotions are coming from. An issue that's completely unrelated to sex, like being stressed about work or frustrated by traffic, can also get in the way.

Unfortunately, many of us get so used to carrying negative emotions that we are no longer aware of them or of the tensions they create in our bodies. This is especially common for men, since a lot of guys have come to believe that having or expressing feelings isn't masculine. But of course men have the same variety of emotions as women, and learning to deal with them works a lot better than pretending they don't happen. Acknowledging and talking about negative emotions clears the air. Not only will you be happier, but it'll make your prostate play much more fun.

Prostate play, in particular, works best when your emotions, your mood, and your body are all on board. Many of the men we've spoken with have said that their experience of prostate massage and anal penetration is different in this way from their usual cock play. After all, lots of guys are able to have intercourse (on the giving end) when they're in a bad mood, have a headache, or have simply had a stressful day. But being penetrated is quite different from doing the penetrating. Some heterosexual men we've spoken with have said that trying the receptive role gave them a much better understanding of how their female partners might not always be interested in receiving. As one guy put it, "There are lots of times when I don't feel like getting fucked but I could totally fuck someone else."

Because of the openness and relaxation required for receiving penetration, many men find that prostate play requires a more specific mental state than cock-centered play. As one of our interviewees put it, "With regard to cock play I am able to get into it even when I have other things bothering me, be they physical, emotional, mental. I can force myself through it, overpower it in a way with the strength of the lust. However, with regard to prostate play, I really need to be clear and calm on all fronts because any of those troubles will distract me from the subtle sensations involved and make it difficult to relax enough to enjoy them." So before you even get started, check in with yourself and see if you're really in the mood. Be honest about whatever is going on for you.

First, check in with your body. How does your body feel? If there is discomfort, are there any steps you can take to remedy it? Maybe a walk around the block? Some stretching to loosen up your lower back? A pain killer for that headache?

Second, check in with your state of mind. Are you angry from that argument with your co-worker? Are you worried about something? Concerned about what might be running through your partner's head? Do you feel rushed? Frustrated with searching for the prostate? If you find that you are having negative emotions come up around prostate play, investigate where they are coming from. Try talking it over with someone you trust, discussing it with your therapist, or hashing it out in a journal. Dealing with the issue is the best way to make it go away.

It can be frustrating when part of you is really eager to explore and another part is holding you back. You may be tempted to try to ignore or push through the negative emotions. But pushing harder can make the situation worse. Any reservations you have are likely to cause more tightening and less pleasure, so don't push. If there's something holding you back, take the time to think it over, look into it, and figure out what it needs. You might want to reread the frequently asked questions about common concerns in chapter 1.

REALISTIC EXPECTATIONS

You may have heard a lot of good things about prostate play, and that may be why you are interested in exploring it. For many who are new to it, it holds a certain mystique as a novel pleasure to discover. Perhaps you've heard grand tales of full-body orgasms and hands-free orgasms that come from prostate massage alone, without any cock play. One prostate toy manufacturer advertises, "Take it from me, guys: prostate massage is the key to achieving the most intense orgasm you will ever experience." Such enthusiastic recommendations are enticing, and it is easy to get caught up in high expectations.

But expectations can be problematic. First, they can distract you from the pleasure at hand. You can become so caught up in what you *want* to happen that you aren't feeling what actually *is* happening at any given moment—or at least, not feeling it as deeply as you could if you weren't so preoccupied. Because you aren't feeling the full depth of the experience, you are missing out on much of what it has to offer. Ironically, this means that your expectations are actually getting in the way of what you are hoping for.

Second, high expectations are easily disappointed. If you are very attached to the idea of having a full-body orgasm on your first try, there's a good chance you will be dissatisfied

> *"Supreme Bliss happens in the moment. Expectations take you out of it into the future."*
>
> —SOMRAJ POKRAS AND JEFFRE TALLTREES

and frustrated if it doesn't happen. Being frustrated is no state of mind in which to experience pleasure. We've heard from men who were really disappointed with their early experiences, and pushed really hard for it the next time. Naturally, they didn't enjoy it then either. Some gave up. Others assumed that their inability to "perform" in this way was due to some inadequacy.

Just as in other types of sex, being too strongly goal-oriented or comparing yourself to what you think someone else is doing can undermine your pleasure. Many men who explore prostate play have amazing experiences. For some, it happens the first time; for others, it takes several tries to find the pleasure in it. Most men will have a mix of experiences—sometimes it's fireworks and other times it's a dud. Then again, some men never get into prostate play, for a variety of reasons. Everyone's experience is unique, and there's no way to predict what it will be like for you.

Don't worry about what this person tells you, or how that person's website describes what prostate play is like for them. All that's important is what you experience. Of course, other people's stories can be helpful when you're starting out—just don't turn them into another goal you have to reach. The point here is to find out what it's like for you.

Try to keep this in mind as you explore. Acknowledge from the start that you don't know how this will go and can't force it to go any particular way. Instead of thinking about what you want to happen, focus on what actually is happening and experience each moment for what it is. There will always be good days and bad days. If you don't get what you want today, there's always tomorrow to try again.

LEARNING TO RECEIVE

Many men find it easier to give pleasure than to receive it. There's a common expectation that a "real man" should always be "in charge," always leading the action. As a result, some men find it difficult to sit back and let their partner take the lead because they worry that it may call their masculinity into question. It's similar to how some men cannot ask for directions: because real men don't admit they are lost. They might drive around for hours laboring under this delusion.

Or, a man may feel that to be a good lover he must always give pleasure to his partner and get his own pleasure from giving it. It's as if he feels it's his responsibility to make his partner feel good, that he's not being a real man if he's not doing that. It's even woven into our language around hetero-sexual sex: men "give" women orgasms, but we rarely hear of women giving men orgasms.

We are totally in favor of men pleasuring their partner when that's what they both want. Problems arise when it becomes not an option but a requirement. It's unfortunate that many men have come to believe that they must always be in charge, in control, that allowing themselves to receive pleasure would be in conflict with their masculinity. These beliefs limit men because they mark a whole range of experiences as off-limits and make it difficult or impossible to live fully free, authentic lives. It means that they don't get to receive, and that they aren't allowing their partners to experience the joy of giving.

We think that one of the best things about allowing your-self to receive pleasure is that it can be a welcome change from always having to be in control. Letting your partner take the lead doesn't mean you have to let go of control completely. You can still ask your partner to change their technique, apply some lube, or shift positions. The role of the top is always there, if you want to pick it up again. If you believe that once you put it down, you lose it forever, we invite you to reconsider that assumption. After all, the fact that you receive penetration today doesn't change your ability to do the penetrating next time.

AROUSAL

What's the difference between a juicy prostate massage and a prostate exam at your doctor's office? Arousal! The state of arousal changes the way all parts of your body experience stimulation. Light caresses can feel electrifying. Your pain tolerance increases. Parts of your body that you may never have considered erogenous zones suddenly become so. Almost any kind of stimulation tends to be more exciting if you are turned on to begin with because you've already got the ball rolling.

Arousal is especially important for prostate play. The prostate, like the female G-spot, fills with fluid during sexual excitement. This swelling not only makes it bigger and easier to locate with fingertips, but also makes it feel different to the receiver. Many men report that the prostate feels most pleasurable if it is massaged when it is very swollen and full of fluid.

This may be different from the way you experience cock stimulation. A lot of men can enjoy having their cock touched even when they are not very turned on or not very erect. They may prefer gentler touches at first, and it may feel different from when they have a full erection, but they can still enjoy touching their cock from the start, without much warm-up.

The prostate is a different kind of tissue. It is the state of arousal, and the accompanying swelling, that makes the prostate receptive to touch. Particularly if you're new to this, massaging your unaroused prostate may feel uninteresting or even uncomfortable, whereas a swollen prostate is likely to yield vastly different and more agreeable sensations.

Not only that, since the prostate engorges and gets bigger when you're turned on, you're much more likely to be able to locate your prostate if you start off with some other kinds of pleasure first, rather than just shoving a finger up there without any kind of turn-on happening. Whether you are solo or with a partner, take time to get excited before you go poking around back there. It may make all the difference.

The Dos and Don'ts of Arousal

- **Do stroke your cock.** For most men, it is the focus of erotic pleasure and can be very useful in making the new sensations of prostate play feel good. You can touch yourself, or your partner can touch you. Particularly if you are new to anal penetration, including this familiar pleasure in the mix is a good idea.

- **Don't ignore the rest of your body!** Pinch your nipples, cup your balls, fondle your ass cheeks, press into your perineum—explore! Ask your partner to give you a full-body massage. Caress as many places as you please, in addition to your cock. As you broaden your erotic focus beyond the cock and into the prostate, don't stop there! The entire body has erogenous potential.

- **Do take breaks from rubbing your cock.** Take some time to lie back and focus on the sensations coming from your prostate—they may be subtle at first and difficult to pick up on. Also, some men find that cock and prostate stimulation together are too much sensation unless they're really turned on. Alternate between cock and prostate to help build toward simultaneous stimulation of both.

- **Don't overdo the cock play.** Prostate sensations can be subtle when you are first learning to feel them, and the force of habit is powerful! For many men, once the cock gets involved it is easy for it to take over the experience. Then the familiar sensations of your cock can override the new, unfamiliar prostate sensations, making it even harder to pick up on them.

- **Do draw it out.** Take your time and go at a relaxed pace. Remember, this isn't a race to the finish line. Many boys learn to masturbate as quickly as possible, and it can be a tough habit to change. But the longer you go, the more time there is for the erotic charge to build. That opens the possibility of more pleasure and a more powerful orgasm.

Take your time and discover what a difference it can make.

- **Don't go too far.** If you get so excited that you feel a sense of urgency, you might want to just get off quickly. Before you know it, you're stroking your way to your habitual penile orgasm. That's just fine if it's what you are in the mood for, but it's not going to help you discover your prostate. If you find yourself speeding up, change what you're doing to allow the arousal to build gradually.

- **Do slow down.** Prostate sensations can be very subtle at first. Slow down and relax while building arousal: this makes it easier to tune in to the new sensations. It may seem counterintuitive—it's common to think that harder, faster strokes are the best way to generate the most sensation. But often this intensity can drown the sensations, and may even cause you to numb out. With slow strokes you can feel more once you learn to tune in. When you've had a bit more practice, you'll probably be able to handle more intensity with your prostate play.

- **Don't overstimulate your prostate.** Many men, when having a hard time reaching a penile orgasm, use rapid strokes on their cock to push themselves over the edge. Well, stroking feverishly at your cock might help you get off that way, but it won't work nearly so well when you are discovering prostate pleasure. The prostate works differently than the penis, so it takes different techniques to make the most of it. If you aren't feeling prostate sensations, hard and fast strokes are likely to drown out the new sensations rather than intensify them. Often this makes the prostate feel uncomfortable or numb. So for now, experiment with slower and lighter touches. Later, once you've learned to feel your prostate, you can see how it likes firmer, quicker strokes.

TO STROKE, OR NOT TO STROKE (YOUR COCK)

A lot of guys include some kind of cock play in their prostate fun. They may find that strokin' it is essential to making prostate play erotic. Some men try anal penetration and prostate massage without cock stimulation and find it to be uncomfortable, overwhelming, or just plain dull. These men tend to get their cock involved every time.

Other men like to put aside their cock while they are exploring their prostate. They find that once the cock is involved, this habitual form of pleasure takes over the experience and dominates the sensory channels, drowning out the prostate sensations. They prefer to sink deeply into the prostate pleasure on its own, magnifying the subtle sensations of the prostate by focusing on them intently to the point where these sensations can feel very powerful indeed. Some men can reach orgasm in this way, from prostate massage alone.

Still other men enjoy both approaches, switching back and

forth from one day to the next as the mood strikes them. That can be a great way to get the best of both worlds.

What should you do? If you are new to prostate massage and anal penetration, we definitely recommend that you include your cock at first. It's a great way to build the arousal, which makes the prostate more receptive and easier to find. If you are used to masturbating with your cock, as most men are, this familiar experience can help your body associate the new sensation with a tried-and-true pleasure. Just be sure to take breaks from the cock play so that you can learn to tune in to your prostate. Try switching back and forth between cock and prostate, then slowly stimulating both at once.

You might also try different masturbation techniques. For example, if you tend to focus on the head of your cock, see what happens if you stroke the whole shaft while playing with your prostate. This helps keep you out of your habitual patterns, especially if you tend to race to the finish line. By giving less attention to the most sensitive areas of your cock, you can give more attention to your prostate. You may find it easier to draw the experience out longer, build more intensity, and discover deeper pleasures.

If you find that switching techniques makes your cock go soft, or if your energy decreases, go back to your usual methods for a while. This should kick-start the arousal and will likely help your prostate become more engorged. Then you can back off a little and return your focus to the prostate. Going back and forth in this way is an excellent method for making your pleasure last longer.

Practice, Practice, Practice

As with any kind of sex, you'll need to experiment a bit and figure out what works for you. Scientists say that an experiment is only a failure if it doesn't answer the questions they're asking. Similarly, if you try something and it doesn't work for you, that doesn't mean it was a failure. Now you know an important piece of information that will help you next time.

Even when you've figured out what works for you, it's possible that you'll need some time to perfect your technique. For example, coordinating the motion of one hand on your cock and the other on a toy can be tricky. That's especially true if the sensations you like on your prostate change when you get more aroused or when you orgasm.

As with any new experience, you will learn more quickly and easily if you practice regularly. Some men make a hobby of prostate exploration, scheduling specific times for practice sessions. Small steps add up and you may be surprised at how quickly your efforts pay off.

It may sound funny to schedule masturbation sessions with yourself, but it's a great way to ensure that you have the time and energy to do it on a regular basis. It doesn't have to feel like a chore—think of it as time that you are devoting to yourself for relaxation and enjoyment. But even if it is scheduled, make sure you only do it when you have the energy for it and you're sincerely in the mood. If it stops being fun, take a vacation from it until your enthusiasm returns.

Try making time for prostate exploration—by yourself or with a partner, using fingers or toys—two to four times per week for a few weeks. As with any practice, doing it frequently yields noticeable changes more quickly. But it's also a good idea to allow some time to pass between play sessions. This gives the erotic energy a chance to build up so you are more charged when the time comes to play.

Regular sessions will get you through the learning curve more quickly, but once you have tapped in to the new sensations, you will likely be able to maintain the ability even if you don't do it as often. Just like riding a bicycle!

REWIRING

For some men, the prostate feels good to the touch from the very first go. Others find prostate sensations very subtle in the beginning. They may feel very little on the first several tries but find that with time and practice they can feel prostate sensations quite powerfully. This is likely due in part to learning which techniques they enjoy most. But we believe there's another factor too. If this is a new kind of stimulation for you, your brain has to *learn* how to interpret it as pleasurable.

Some have called this the "rewiring" process. When you stimulate the prostate, or any part of the body, nerves pick up the sensation and send signals to your brain. Then the brain—the one true pleasure organ—interprets those signals and decides whether to register the stimuli as pleasure, pain, or something else. If a type of stimulation is unfamiliar, the brain might not know how to interpret it at first. This means that the first few tries might feel different from later experiences.

This is very common when someone tries something new.

Think of it as like acquiring a taste for liquor or for a new kind of food, or like starting a new workout routine such as jogging: it may be challenging at first, but if you do it regularly, it starts to feel good. This can also happen the first time a person uses a sex toy. Maybe it doesn't do much the first time you try it, but you might enjoy it more after a few tries.

We think this might explain why some men who are looking for their prostate (and, for that matter, some women who are looking for their G-spot) may not feel much pleasure on the first few attempts, even if they are touching the right places. You are learning how to experience a new sensation in a new way.

OPEN TO THE SENSATION

As you explore the sensations of your prostate, it helps to approach the experience with a feeling of curiosity about what you might experience, rather than attachment to having a particular kind of experience. Pay attention and see what unique sensations arise. You are learning how to pick up on sensations that may not be familiar to you.

Most of the time, we walk around without really noticing everything going on. We're surrounded by so many stimuli yelling for our attention, it makes sense that we usually tune out most of them. But this habit of tuning out can make it harder to notice the quieter things which we are used to ignoring.

You might be surprised at how much you can pay attention to with a little practice. For example, right now, without looking up from this text, notice how much you can see in your peripheral vision. There are colors and shapes that you are visually processing but your conscious attention was not tuning in to.

What about the sounds? Can you hear cars driving by? People talking on the street? The refrigerator humming in the next room?

Now feel your body—are you warm or cool? Are your muscles relaxed or tense? You might notice that chronic pain in your shoulder, or perhaps your leg is falling asleep? In looking for your prostate, you are applying this same curious, open attention to your own pleasure sensations.

You may find that it helps if you slow down. As Mantak Chia put it, "Often men go from erection to ejaculation like race cars, without taking the time to notice, let alone enjoy, the sights along the way." If you're rushing to the finish line, odds are that you'll miss out on a lot of what prostate play can offer. Take it easy and relax. You'll have more fun, and when you do reach your orgasm, it'll probably be better for it.

If you can let go of your expectations, slow down, and pay attention, with practice you will be able to tune in to your prostate. Over time, it'll get easier and the sensations will get stronger.

Breathe

Telling someone to breathe is a deceptively simple instruction. Breathing doesn't sound like a big deal. It sounds so easy—just breathe!

It sounds so simple, in fact, that many people write it off

as unimportant and don't bother paying attention to it. But the way you breathe actually makes a big difference in the pleasure you can experience during sex.

One of the most common sexual patterns we've seen for men is the tendency to hold their breath during sex. Sometimes it's because they learned to masturbate in secret and as quickly as possible to avoid getting caught. Making noise was a big no-no, so holding the breath became a habit. But whatever the reason for it, holding your breath may not be the best way to tap into prostate sensations.

Imagine an athlete running down a track or a football field. Does he hold his breath? Of course not! Breathing fuels his ability to run, so the better his breathing, the better the running. And that goes for prostate play too.

When you take deep breaths, you're bringing more oxygen into your bloodstream—that means more of what your body needs to run the pleasure machine. Breathing deeply helps you feel more of the sensations and lets the sexual energy flow more smoothly throughout the body. That means more pleasure for you.

The importance of breathing came up again and again in our survey. A lot of men favor long, slow, deep breaths when they do prostate play. Consciously breathing in this way will help the body relax and settle in to the sensations.

You can also try 10–15 short, quick breaths (sometimes called "breath of fire") to raise your energy, followed by some long, deep breaths to spread it around. Imagine your sexual energy rising up your body from your prostate until it reaches your head. Can you breathe it all the way up? If not, try for a little more each time. You may be surprised at how much better it makes things feel.

PC Muscle Tone

There is an important muscle in the pelvic floor that supports the genital and anal structures. It is shaped like a *V* with the wide end in front and the point in back. This muscle is called the *pubococcygeus*, or PC for short, because it runs between the pubic bone (located just above your penis) and the coccyx or tailbone (the bottom tip of the spine). Some use the term *PC muscle group* to refer to the PC plus some other pelvic floor muscles that usually work in tandem, such as the anal sphincters.

In women, contracting the PC muscle causes the vagina to squeeze. In men, because the muscle surrounds the rectum and the bulb of the penis, it contracts to help ejaculation during orgasm. If you squeeze this muscle when your penis is erect, it will cause the cock to bounce upward.

The tone of the PC group is important to sexual response in both men and women. These muscles twitch during the buildup of arousal and contract rhythmically during orgasm. Getting your PC group in shape can make orgasms feel more intense, make anal penetration easier, and decrease the refractory period—the resting time after ejaculation before you can get erect again. You can get your PCs in shape by doing Kegel exercises. This is the practice of squeezing and releasing the PC muscle group in isolation, without flexing anything else.

A toned muscle isn't one that's tight all the time. In fact, for a lot of men, the problem isn't that the muscle is too weak, but rather that it can't relax. If you spend a lot of time sitting or driving, and especially if you tend to be stressed out, odds are that your PC muscle is too tight. When the muscle is toned, it can both tighten and relax. That's what we're aiming for.

Finding the PC muscle is easy. The next time you have to urinate, sit down on the toilet. Start peeing and then stop the flow of urine. The muscle you use to do this is the PC muscle. Now try flexing that muscle without moving your stomach, butt, or thighs. If you can do this, you are flexing the muscle in isolation, which is important for increasing its tone. Once you've found it and learned to flex it in isolation, you can do these exercises anytime, anywhere, because the action is not externally visible.

There are a few basic ways to do Kegels, listed below. Start off doing five of each and ramp up until you can do sets of 15 or 20. Don't overdo it—you can make the PC muscle sore, just like any other workout.

- Squeeze/release on a one count. Hold the muscle firm on a one count and then release it on a one count.

- Squeeze/release on a two count. Same as above, only a bit slower, which lets you tune into what you're doing.

- Squeeze/release on a four count. In this one, firm the muscle for a four count, hold it for a four count, release over a four count, and relax for a four count.

- Butterflies. This time, firm the muscle quickly and

let go. As it releases and before it fully relaxes, do it again. Afterward, let it fully relax for an equal amount of time.

Be sure to let the muscle fully relax between squeezes, or at the end of a set of butterflies. Muscles need to rest in order to build strength. Start off with just a few repetitions per set and increase as you gain more ability—just like going to the gym.

As your PC muscle gains tone, you'll probably find that you have more control over your anus, so it will become easier to relax it in order to receive penetration. You might also discover that your orgasms feel more intense. That's because when your PC muscle has more endurance and strength, it is able to contract harder, longer, and more repeatedly. If you don't notice a change, the difference may have come on slowly. But after doing the exercises for a few months, if you suddenly stop, you'll probably be able to tell the difference. Fortunately, if you lose your PC muscle tone, you can always get it back by repeating the exercises.

TWO APPROACHES: TANTRA AND FANTASY

We want to discuss briefly two different schools of thought regarding the pursuit of pleasure. One is Tantra, the other is fantasy. These are two very popular and very different approaches to sex play.

The Tantric approach to sexuality uses a number of techniques such as breathing exercises and vocalizations to get more deeply in touch with the sensations of the body and the present moment. It is a fusing of sexuality and spirituality in which every moment can be felt as sacred. Some are put off by Tantra because it can seem weird or hippie-dippie, but once you get over the initial self-consciousness, it has quite a lot to offer. In Tantric sex, you bring meditation into the bedroom and learn to be more present to what is happening in your body in each moment, so you can feel your sensations as though they are magnified. Quite a lot of men find that a Tantric approach, which emphasizes relaxing and getting into the body, is very useful in exploring the prostate. To go in depth into Tantric technique is beyond the scope of this book, but see the Resources for suggestions of Tantra guides.

The fantasy approach, on the other hand, is less about zooming in on your sensations and more about focusing on sexy ideas, images, or story lines in your imagination. Fantasizing during masturbation or sex can bring up a great deal of erotic charge and can jump-start your excitement even before any touch occurs. You can let your imagination run wild as you explore and see what fantasy images and scenarios turn you on. If you find that you are turned on by a fantasy you consider inappropriate, you are not alone. Everyone has fantasies, and many of the juicier ones—the ones that really turn you on—involve some kind of "inappropriate" behavior. This can cause us to feel guilty, confused, or ashamed and wonder if there is something wrong with us. But being turned on by a story in your head doesn't mean that you want to enact it in real life. As long as you are clear on that distinction, you are free to enjoy whatever fantasies turn you on. For inspiration, consult erotic fiction or pornography, or check out Violet Blue's *The Ultimate Guide to Sexual Fantasy*.

It's worth noting that the fantasy approach to pleasure, in which you concentrate on hot images or story lines in your imagination, is very different from the Tantric approach, which seeks to focus all your attention on what is actually happening each moment. Yet both approaches are popular among men who get into prostate play. We don't suggest that either approach is the right way, or the best way. If you are so inclined, we would encourage you to try both.

WHAT YOU MIGHT FEEL

You might experience many different sensations as you look for your prostate. Here are a few common ones.

"Gotta pee"

This is a good sign! Lots of men get the "gotta pee" sensation when they first feel pressure on the prostate, so this probably means that you are in the right spot. Continue to gently explore that area. Take a few deep breaths and allow yourself to feel it rather than fighting against it. The sensation of needing to urinate should pass, often replaced by pleasure.

WHY DO I FEEL LIKE I HAVE TO PEE?

Many men, when they first feel pressure on their prostate, get a feeling like they have to pee. This "gotta pee" feeling is common in G-spot play as well.

Of course, you probably don't really have to pee. The prostate surrounds the urethra, directly below the bladder, so when the bladder is full, it exerts pressure on the prostate. When you get that "gotta pee" feeling during prostate massage, your body is simply taking the pressure sensation to mean what it usually means: a full bladder to be emptied.

If you are worried about peeing during your play, you can put yourself at ease by emptying your bladder beforehand. Then you may find it easier to relax into the sensation. You can also lay down some towels or play in the bathtub. Rest assured that, in the absence of an infection, it's safe to come into contact with urine.

The Urge to Come

Some men ejaculate spontaneously when their prostate is massaged, especially if it's one of their first few tries. Normally, the feeling of pressure in your prostate coincides with ejaculation: fluid fills the prostatic urethra right before it is sent along its way out the cock. If you feel the urge to come during your exploration and you are ready to end the session, by all means go ahead. If you'd like to continue playing, hold still and breathe slowly to allow the sensation to pass.

Discomfort

Some tenderness and mild discomfort is common when you are new to anal penetration and prostate massage. This is a sign that your body is getting used to this new form of stimulation. You may be a little sore the next day, so take it easy. Over time, this tenderness goes away. For now, don't press any harder than what is comfortable. Pushing through your discomfort is unlikely to bring pleasure. Instead, go softly and build up slowly. Don't try to force your body to experience a pleasure that it isn't ready for. If it starts to hurt, or if it stops being fun, call it a day and try again another time.

Numbness

It's not unusual for a man to feel nothing at all when pressing directly on his prostate. This may mean that he is not aroused enough, or simply that he has not yet awakened the sensation of his prostate. If it's a new kind of stimulation for you, your brain will need to figure out how to receive it. It may take a while for it to be interpreted as pleasure. If this happens, continue what you're doing and be sure to take slow deep breaths. Take a break and repeat the massage in a minute— sometimes it feels completely different when you try it again. This often works better than plugging away at it until you are sore. Try putting down your cock while rubbing the spot—the familiar sensations of cock stimulation can sometimes override the new, subtle sensations of prostate massage.

Pleasure

It just might feel good! Yes, crazy idea—it just might feel like a deep, aching pleasure. If that happens, good for you! Relax, take your time, and enjoy it.

SOURCE OF QUOTE

Somraj Pokras and Jeffre TallTrees, *Tantric Male Multiple G-Spot Orgasm,* e-book (Tantra at Tahoe, 2003), 102.

7

FIND IT:
LOCATING THE GLAND

In the previous chapter we laid the foundation for feeling your prostate sensations. Now it's time to physically locate the gland. We've divided this chapter into sections for men who are looking for their own prostate and those who are looking for a partner's. People who are doing this with a partner may also find the information in the solo section useful.

Even if you plan to do this with a partner, we think starting off solo makes a lot of sense. When you do it alone, you don't have to worry about a partner's expectations, concerns, or reactions. You can also go at your own pace. After some solo practice, you'll be better equipped to tell a partner what you like. In our experience, that makes it a lot easier.

SET THE SCENE

Preparing for your exploration only takes a short while and can make a big difference in your experience. Getting things ready in advance means fewer distractions while you play, so you'll be better able to focus. Whether you are exploring solo or with a partner, take time beforehand to get yourself and your play space ready.

- **Make time.** Set aside at least one hour or more during which you have nothing to do except relax and explore. More time is better if you can swing it. Budget your energy—pick a time when you will be awake and will have energy to spare. Make sure you've eaten within the past few hours so that you won't run out of steam.

- **Minimize distractions.** Find a time when you will have privacy. Turn off the phone and lock the bedroom door. If you are concerned that someone might hear you, play some music.

- **Set up.** Gather all your supplies so you have them handy. You don't want to have to get up and go searching for something in the middle of your exploration. Lay out a towel to catch lube drips and a second, "discard" towel so you have a place to put used gloves and toys when you are done with them.

- **Clean and shine.** Take a shower or bath to wash up and let go of the day. If that's not an option, use hypoallergenic wipes to ensure that the outside of the anus is clean. Make sure your fingernails are filed short and smooth, with no snags or sharp corners. Remember that the anus is as sensitive as the lips on your face, so run your nails along your lips to check for rough spots that may need to be trimmed. Be sure to remove any rings before penetration happens!

- **Empty the tank.** Go to the bathroom before getting started. Since prostate play sometimes makes you feel like you need to pee, knowing that your bladder is empty helps you relax and enjoy yourself. If you have regular bowel movements, time your anal play for after you've had one, and you won't need to worry about having to take a shit during your playtime. If it will help you feel more comfortable, give yourself an enema. (For enema tips, see chapter 4, Hygiene.)

PROSTATE EXPLORATION CHECKLIST

__ Lube
__ Gloves
__ Pillows
__ Towels

__ Wet wipes
__ Toys
__ Condoms for toys
__ A glass of water

SOLO EXPLORATION: LOCATE THE PROSTATE

One of the best ways to find your prostate is with your fingers. For some men, this is simply not physically possible. Others can actually get themselves off this way. Those who have good flexibility and long arms and fingers will be at an advantage. Due to the awkwardness of the position, you may not be able to continue the search for very long. But if you can maintain the position long enough to locate the gland with your fingers, you'll have a better idea of where to direct a toy or a partner later. You may not manage to rub yourself all the way to a prostate orgasm, but simply getting familiar with the sensation is a step along the way.

If you can't quite reach the spot, enlist the aid of a toy! Many toys work great for prostate play. Check out chapter 11, Toys, for more information.

Solo Exploration Positions

The positions involved in rubbing your prostate may put strain on your wrist and perhaps some other parts as well. Listen to your body—if something starts to hurt, take a break. Do some other kind of stimulation for a few minutes and then return to your prostate exploration. Or call it a day—it's not worth giving yourself a sore wrist. Try these positions:

- Lie on your back, with your hips propped up on a pile of pillows. Put pillows under your upper back as well so you're curled up with your back rounded. (This will increase your reach.) Your knees are bent with feet flat on the bed, or your legs are drawn in toward your chest.

- Squat down with your knees wide and hips low to the ground.

- Get on your hands and knees, with your head lowered to the ground.

- Lie on your side with your bottom leg straight and the top leg bent with knee drawn up, resting on a pillow.

- Stand up with one foot elevated on a stool. Do this near the wall so you can use it for balance.

Reaching for It

There are two approaches you could take to massaging your prostate: reach down between your legs, or reach around back.

Reach down

This is the most common approach, and it works well with any of the positions described above. Once in position, reach down between your legs, insert one or two fingers (using lube, of course!), and curl your fingers toward the front of the body, as if you were trying to reach the deep end of your cock with your fingertips. This makes for a dramatic flexion of the wrist and fingers.

Reach around back

This approach tends to work best in positions where one leg is up and the other down, such as standing with one leg on a stool or lying on your side with one leg drawn up.

Once you are in position, twist your upper body toward the leg that is lifted up, and reach the same arm behind your back. Now try inserting your thumb. If your thumb is long enough, you can reach the prostate with the pad of your thumb. You can now explore the gland by curling the thumb or shifting it from side to side.

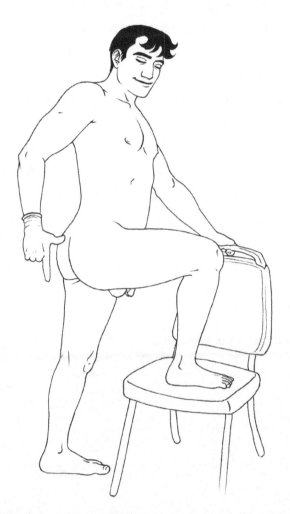

Illustration 3. Solo Massage Position: Reach around Back

FEELING FOR IT: GUIDED SOLO EXPLORATION

So, you are feeling frisky and ready to explore! You have set up your space, everything you need is handy, and you've gotten yourself nicely aroused. Time to look for the prostate. Here's what to do.

If you wish, put on a glove. Put a dab of lube on your fingertip and rub it on the anal opening. Massage it lightly to relax the sphincters and get the area warmed up. Take your time here—don't rush past this step. The more relaxed you are, the easier and more fun it will be.

When you are ready, insert a finger slowly. If you are also playing with your cock, you may want to pause for a moment—stroking your cock can cause the PC muscles to contract, which feels good but makes anal penetration more difficult.

Be sure to follow the anal guidelines listed in chapter 5, Penetration 101. Don't be rough or forceful—it'll just make your anus tighten down more. Take your time. Breathe deep, long breaths and don't forget to exhale!—that's the relaxing part of the breath. Once your finger is inside, hold still for a moment. How long? Until the penetration feels comfortable and movement feels welcome.

LOSS OF ERECTION

It is very common for men to lose their erection when penetrated. The reasons for this aren't totally clear. In some cases, it may be the result of anxiety about being penetrated. In others, it may simply be that the man's attention has shifted to a different part of his body. Since the pelvic muscles relax to accommodate penetration, this may allow blood to drain out of the penis, causing it to go soft. Try not to be attached to having a hard-on the whole time; it may come and go throughout the exploration. In the meantime, you can still stroke your cock, and chances are the nerve endings will still be very responsive. Arousal, orgasm, and ejaculation are all possible without a hard-on.

BUTT PLUGS HELP

Butt plugs can be very helpful in prepping the ass for fingers. If you have a small one, insert it and let it sit for a while before you begin the finger exploration.

Butt plugs are designed to go in and stay put, so you can leave one in while you do other kinds of play. Meanwhile, it helps your ass relax and get used to being penetrated. Later, when you are ready for fingers, it's as if you had them in the whole time—except that you didn't have to hold still all the while, and your hands were free to do other things. Since your ass has been receiving an object all along, it's likely to be well prepared for the gentle motions of your finger exploration.

As your finger slides in, you first pass through two rings of muscle, the anal sphincters. If you contract your PC muscles, you can feel the sphincters tighten around your finger. Try to contract and release several times—this helps you gain awareness and control of the sphincters. Move deeper and you will notice that just beyond this muscular passage, known as the anal canal, the space feels softer and more open; it curves and then flattens out more or less parallel to the front of the body. This is the rectum. Now the search begins.

Find the Shape

The prostate can be felt through the front wall of the rectum. After you pass through the muscular anal canal and enter the soft rectum, slide your fingers along the front wall of the rectal tissue. At first it feels soft when you press it, but as you go a little deeper it will feel firm. Feel along the front wall to see if you can make out the form of the prostate with your fingers. The more aroused you are, the more swollen it will be. And the more swollen it is, the larger and more rounded it becomes, so it is easier to find.

The prostate is shaped roughly like a sphere, but you can only touch the back side of it because the rest of it is embedded in the surrounding tissue of the pelvis. Remember the plum image? Imagine a plum that is about three-quarters buried in sand, so that you can only feel a portion of it. You are only feeling one face of a sphere.

On the surface of the prostate where you are touching, there is an indentation running vertically down the middle. In some men, this indentation may not be very well defined—

especially in older men who may have benign prostatic hyper-trophy (BPH), a condition in which the prostate grows larger, which can alter its shape. However, in many men this midline indentation is very tangible and you can rest your finger in this gentle groove. If you slide your finger to the right or left of the midline, you can feel that the prostate forms a rounded lobe on each side—again, very much like a plum. If you continue a little further outward, you will feel where each lobe rounds off and disappears into the body. The rest of the gland is buried too deep to be felt. The term *gutters* has been used to describe the space beyond each lobe, where you can settle your finger on either side of the prostate.

The texture of the prostate has been described as "spongy" or "rubbery." Usually, it feels more firm than most of the surrounding tissue, though if there is a lot of pelvic muscle tension, it can be harder to make out. Press a finger to the tip of your nose, and another to the soft skin of your cheek. This nicely illustrates the way it feels when you press the rectal wall at the prostate, versus pressing the rectal wall to the side of or deeper than the prostate.

Remember, the prostate can be felt *through* the front wall of the rectum, not *on* the rectal wall. So the prostate will feel more firm when you apply pressure, but as you slide your fingers along the rectal wall, the surface texture at the pros-tate will feel identical to other parts of the rectum: smooth and soft with gentle folds.

Explore the Sensations

If you can make out the shape of the gland, great! Now you can explore how it feels. Press against it as though you were reaching for your cock from the inside—remember that the prostate is located just behind the base of the cock. Try stimulating different areas of the gland separately: the deep end, the right and left lobes, the central valley.

The prostate will probably not register light caresses—it responds to pressure. However, there's a point at which too much pressure becomes uncomfortable or painful. Resist the temptation to dig in hard in the hope that it will make you feel more. Chances are, it will only make you feel *more discomfort*. When you are new to massage, the prostate may feel a little tender for the first few sessions, but less so with practice. Look for a happy medium: firm, but not too firm. Avoid digging in with your fingertips—that is likely to hurt.

Here are a few suggestions for things you can try. Do each stroke several times before moving on to the next, and pay attention to how it feels.

Reach down between the legs

- Hold your finger in one spot and press and hold for a second, then release the pressure and be still for a second. Repeat this several times over the same spot.

- Reach for the deep end (the top of the gland) and tug downward on it as if you were trying to pull it out.

- Slide your fingertip down the surface of the gland from top to bottom.

Reach around from behind

- If using your thumb, curl it or swivel it from side to side.

Pay attention to how it feels. If it feels uncomfortable, don't press so hard. If you find that rubbing a certain area creates a different sensation from the surrounding landscape, you may be on the right track. Continue to play with that area and see what happens. In particular, pay attention to places that feel tingly or pleasurable, or that make you feel like you want to come or need to pee. You may find that when you first massage a location it feels unremarkable, but after going over that area a second time you begin to notice something different.

"I Can't Find It"

You might not be able to make out the form of the prostate at first, and that's fine. You can still explore for it. Simply reach your finger or thumb as deep as you can inside the rectum, and apply pressure through the front wall, pressing toward your belly. Keep your finger or thumb on this spot and maintain the pressure for a few seconds, then release for a few seconds; repeat several times. Now withdraw your finger slightly—just a half-inch—and do the same press-and-release exercise, focusing on that spot. Continue all the way down the front wall until you reach the end of the rectum, where it meets the tight muscular tube formed by the anal sphincters. The idea is to explore the whole front wall, starting as far in as you can reach and slowly working your way down toward the anal canal. When you finish a set, reinsert your finger and repeat from the beginning. You can also do a set slightly right or left of center to focus on the right or left lobe, but make sure you are always pressing the front wall.

This kind of top-to-bottom rubdown will work well if you are reaching between your legs, but it might be more difficult to get various depths of penetration in the reach-behind positions. If you're reaching behind, just massage where you can reach, moving slightly to the right or left if you can and slightly up and down if you can.

Hopefully, you will find a place that feels different from the surrounding tissue. As you continue, the pressure you apply may contribute to the swelling of the gland and soon you may find that the form becomes more clearly defined and recognizable. After a few sets, if you still can't make out the shape of the prostate, withdraw your finger to give your wrist a break. Focus on other stimulation to keep your energy up. You may find the prostate to be more swollen and sensitive when you return and look again.

Be sure to save a little wrist strength for the moment of orgasm. Even if you have had little success so far in the exploration, having a finger on the prostate at the moment of climax can feel amazing! You may find that the orgasm feels broader, deeper, more full-bodied, or more intense than what you are used to from your cock alone.

Also, because the prostate swells dramatically just before

and during ejaculation, it's easier to make out its shape with your fingertips. If you weren't sure where it was before, you'll know for sure afterward!

BLOOD IN THE SEMEN

Sometimes a man may find trace amounts of blood in his semen after ejaculating, giving the fluid a pinkish tinge. This occasionally happens after a prostate massage. It can be quite alarming, but it is actually very common, and not only in the context of prostate massage. Often it is only a burst blood vessel.[14] This is the same thing that happens when you get a bruise, or when you blow your nose and there's a little blood on the tissue—nothing to be concerned about.

If you find a faintly pinkish tinge of blood in your semen after a prostate massage, wait a few days before repeating the massage, and maybe go easier on the pressure next time, particularly if it feels tender. In the vast majority of cases, the problem goes away on its own and isn't a cause for concern.[15] If it does not go away within a week, or if you have other troublesome symptoms, it may be time to see a doctor.

PARTNERED EXPLORATION: LOCATE THE PROSTATE

Although solo play has its advantages, there are many reasons why you might like to invite a partner to help you. If you have a good erotic connection, simply having your partner present might make it feel more charged than if you were on your own. Chances are they will be able to reach your prostate more effectively than you can, which means better stimulation for you. Because you won't be straining to reach it yourself, you'll also be more comfortable, so the exploration can go a little longer. And, in the absence of pretzel-like positioning and distracting physical strain, you'll be better able to relax and focus on the sensations at hand.

This section contains tips for exploring the prostate with a partner. Once again, the purpose is to locate it. What to do once you find it is covered in chapter 9, Prostate Massage.

Communication Before, During, After

Open communication is a major key to successful exploration with a partner. Lots of different things can happen, so being able to talk about whatever comes up will make this easier. Due to the sensitivity of the anal area, pleasure can switch quickly to pain because of insufficient lube or involuntary tightening of the anal sphincters. And because anal play is a big taboo for some people, big emotions can come up without warning. Good things can happen too—like immense pleasure as your partner suddenly finds the right spot. So tell your partner about it! Let them know what's going on for you: the good, the bad, and the neutral.

Some people are hesitant to give their partner feedback during sex. There's a widespread myth that if the connection between you is real, your partner will just intuitively know how to please you. Or that asking for what you want makes the experience less spontaneous, or less authentic. And some people are afraid of hurting their partner's feelings with negative feedback.

But the fact is, no matter how well tuned in to each other you are, no one is a mind reader. It isn't always possible for them to know exactly what you are experiencing, even if they guess right some of the time. Telling your partner what you want and what you don't want doesn't mean your partner is doing a poor job, or you aren't enjoying it, or the sex is less "real"—it means you are taking responsibility for your desires and helping your partner fulfill their desire—which is to make you feel good.

Those who are not in the habit of talking openly during sex may find that it feels awkward at first. As with any new skill, there is a learning curve. But with practice, it will feel perfectly natural. Here are some tips for good communication:

Get started on the right foot

Don't wait to talk until you have something that needs to be voiced. Begin each session by telling your partner what you would like to do ("I'd love to try out a bent-over position today") and what you aren't interested in ("I don't think I'm ready for more than one finger"). These are only predictions; you might change your mind during play. But saying what you want now when you are fully clothed will make it much easier to say what you want later when you have a finger up your bottom.

Talk about concerns

If you have any nagging anxieties about what's going to happen during your play, talk it over with your partner. If you catch it in time, try to do it before the clothes come off. It may help you both relax if you agree in advance that either one of you can stop at any time for any reason.

Sometimes concerns come up during play, and often we don't want to tell our partners because we'd rather not interrupt the flow of the sex. But chances are that if you don't talk about it, your concern will continue looping through your head. At that point, the thought itself has interrupted the flow of sex, making you distracted and inhibited. Call a time-out and tell your partner what you're worried about so you can talk it over and move on. Here are some examples:

"I'm worried that it's going to smell."

"I'm concerned that it's going to be messy."

"I keep thinking it's going to hurt, and that makes me tense up."

Give positive feedback

When your partner does something that works well, let them know. This will clue them in to what you like. Plus, if you give helpful suggestions or negative feedback later ("Ouch! That hurts!"), it's less likely to feel to your partner like they're doing a bad job. Keep it balanced in the positive direction with lots of comments such as "I like that" and "It feels good when you…"

Some relationship experts say that couples need a balance of five positive interactions to one negative in order to keep things flowing smoothly. While we don't think you need to keep track obsessively, this advice does highlight the fact that when you have a foundation of positive feedback, it makes it easier to give and receive the occasional helpful suggestion.

Ask your partner to describe the action

We're not suggesting that you request a play-by-play. But if anything feels especially amazing—or unpleasant—ask your partner to describe what they were doing so you can ask for it to happen (or not happen) again. There's a big difference between saying "I'd like it if you did that amazing thing you did that time" and "I'd like it if you used two fingers in a circular motion on my prostate, like you did that time."

Tell your partner if it hurts

You should never put up with pain when exploring anal penetration and prostate massage. Even if you are capable of tolerating it, it's not a good idea: you could hurt the delicate tissue that lines the anus and rectum. Small, painful tears are a common result of overzealous anal play. Much worse could happen if you are very careless, especially if your senses are dulled with substances or if you are playing with unsafe objects.

Despite myths to the contrary, it isn't likely that the pain will suddenly give way to pleasure. Your partner wants you to feel good, but not at the expense of putting up with pain. Tell them if they are doing something that hurts, so they can stop doing it.

Give direction

"More pressure...a little slower... Right there!" Only you know what you are feeling inside your body, so clue your partner in. It may be helpful to distinguish between "stop" and "hold still," since "stop" could mean either "halt the motion" or "pull out."

Sometimes your partner may ask you how you want it and you won't know. In these cases you can always say, "I don't know. Let's just keep exploring."

Enjoy the afterglow

When the exploration is over, focus on the positive. Tell your partner what you enjoyed and how much fun you had. Any ideas for how it might be better next time? Anything you didn't like? Tuck it in your pocket and save it for another conversation. It's important to share these thoughts, but now is not the time. If you share them now, it can easily over-shadow the good feelings and leave your partner with a sour impression.

For Partners of Men: Tips for Givin' It to Him
Talk him through it

Doctors know the importance of telling the patient what to expect. Instead of letting your partner wonder if you are suddenly going to shove a third finger up there, put him at ease by telling him what you are doing at every step of the way: "Now I'm just teasing the hole. I won't go in until you say you're ready... Ready now? Okay, here's one finger, nice and slow..." Exploring new and potentially charged kinds of sex can be enough to put someone on edge without the added stress of wondering what's coming and when.

Ask for permission

You should ask for permission before you enter him—every time. This reassures him that he is in control of what happens to his ass, and that you only want to give him what he wants to receive. It feels less like an invasion and more like he is inviting you in. This is essential for reassuring an anxious newbie, but even if you've been in his ass a million times, asking permission is still a great way to build a sense of trust between you and your partner. A simple "Are you ready?" can make a big difference.

This, or that?

If he's new at this, he may not yet have discovered what he likes, so it may be hard for him to tell you what he wants. In such cases, instead of asking "What do you want?" you might try the eye doctor's strategy: "Which is better—one, or two?" Do two different kinds of strokes and then ask, "What feels better right now: this, or that?" Bear in mind that while option A feels better now, option B might feel better in 10 minutes.

Listen to his concerns

Sometimes during sex we have anxieties or concerns that don't seem to make sense, and we may feel that we shouldn't be having them. But they come up in spite of all our logical reasoning, and telling ourselves that they shouldn't be there often only makes them worse. Be sensitive toward any concerns that your partner shares with you, even if you don't "get it." We all have reasons for feeling the way we do, even if those reasons aren't always clear, and it's important to be respectful of your partner's concerns.

Let him call the shots

If he asks you to do it in a certain way, and if it isn't a problem for you, try to accommodate the request. He's already in a very vulnerable position and it can put him more at ease to show him that he is still in control of what's happening to his body.

Don't push

If he says to stop, halt the motion immediately. If he asks you to withdraw, do so promptly—but slowly, so you don't hurt him. Don't try to convince him to keep going. You may want to give him a perfect experience and it can be disappointing if that doesn't happen. But don't push it—when he's done, he's done. You may feel *so close* to getting him there, but if he has lost interest, it doesn't matter how skillful you are—his heart isn't in it. Call it a day and try again next time.

Tread carefully

If you are a female partner of a straight man or a male partner of a guy who is usually a top, be extra careful in the approach that you take: you may unintentionally step on a land mine. Men who are used to being the giver may feel defensive at first about allowing themselves to take the receptive role. Watch for signs of inner conflict, and be very gentle if you bring it up. Unless you have negotiated specifically for a power exchange, do not act as though you are dominating him; this can trigger difficult thoughts and feelings for some.

Positions for Partnered Exploration

There are a lot more options for prostate play with a partner than solo. You'll need to experiment a bit to figure out which positions are most comfortable for both of you. Here are some great ones to start with.

On his back

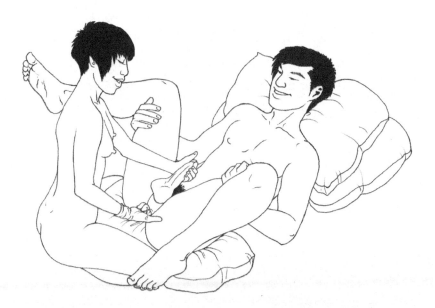

Illustration 4. Partner Massage Position: On His Back

- When he's on his back, with his legs apart, you can sit between his knees. This position lets you maintain eye contact and can help him relax his abdominal muscles, especially if he props his knees up with pillows or supports them with his hands. It may be more comfortable for both of you if there's a pillow under his hips, because that helps him stay relaxed and gives you easier access.

• Try having him lie on the edge of the bed with his knees pulled up to his chest. You can stand on the floor at the side of the bed and have maximum access.

• If you're fortunate enough to have a sling or sex swing, that will work great. (See chapter 12, Anal Sex and Strap-on Fucking, for more information about slings.) Adjust the height so that you can stand or sit in front of the sling and have your arm resting at a comfortable level for penetration.

From behind

- Hands and knees. He's on his hands and knees or on his elbows and knees. You can sit or kneel behind him or at his side.

- Flat on his belly. Prop his ass up with a pillow for better access to his anus. As a variation, you could sit on the bed or on a couch and have him lie across your lap as if you were going to give him an over-the-knee spanking.

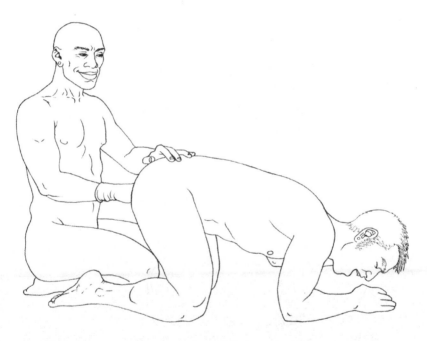

Illustration 5. Partner Massage Position: Hands and Knees

Other positions

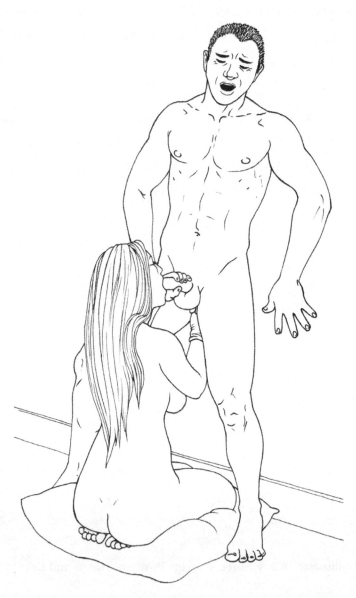

Illustration 6: Partner Massage Position: Standing at Wall

- Standing at wall. Try having him stand up while you kneel on the floor and reach up between his legs or reach around behind him. This is great for combining with hand jobs and blow jobs. Just be mindful of lube drips on slippery floors!

- Pile driver. This position is a bit more strenuous than many of the others: it puts a lot of weight on your neck and shoulders. For that reason, this position should not be attempted by anyone who is not in very good physical shape—in terms of both strength and flexibility. If you decide to try it, be extra careful of your body: if you start to feel signs of physical strain, come out slowly and carefully. Avoid jerky motions with your neck.

To get into this position, lie on your back, then bring your hips up so that they are over your head with your knees coming to rest by your face. Then place your hands under your back to prop it up, so most of your weight rests on your shoulders. This can put strain on the neck, so do it on a soft surface like a bed. It's also a good idea to do some gentle stretching beforehand, and avoid jerking your neck around once you are in position. It helps to position yourself so that a wall is a foot or so from your head so that you can prop your feet against it.

You can also try this on one end of a sturdy couch: sit lightly on the arm of the couch, facing outward, then lean back until you are lying on the couch with your ass still up on the arm. Your head should be lower than your hips and your feet up in the air. To get out of this position, simply roll sideways off the couch (slowly and carefully).

Guided Partner Exploration

When you are looking for your partner's prostate, you are always pressing toward the front of his body. If he is lying on his belly, your palm faces down. If he is lying on his back, your palm faces up.

The length of your fingers will affect your technique. If your fingers are short (say, 3 inches in length) you will need to reach as deep as you can to contact the deep end of the prostate with your fingertips. And in order to get that deep, you'll probably need to press in a little, stretching the muscles of the pelvic floor in the process. This means that if his muscles are very tight, you will have a hard time getting in deep enough to contact the whole surface of the gland. If your fingers are longer (say, 4 inches) this will be less of an issue.

See if you can make out the form of the prostate. Take a minute to get familiar with the landscape. Try to identify the midline, with the two lobes rising on either side. Feel where the gland ends on the right and left sides. Curl your fingertip around the top.

If you are able to feel the prostate, experiment with gently massaging it. Try sliding down it from top to bottom, or curling your fingers around the deep end of the gland and tugging downward. (More in-depth techniques are described in chapter 9, Prostate Massage.) Go very slowly and not too hard. Be mindful that you are using the pads of your fingers (not the tips) and that you are not digging in with your fingernails.

Start with a light pressure and build slowly to a moderate pressure, but be sure to check in with him that it isn't too much pressure. Take breaks between sets so that the prostate doesn't become overstimulated and numb out or start to feel uncomfortable. You can either take the pressure off the prostate while keeping your finger inside him, or remove your finger, as he prefers.

If you are not sure that you have located the gland, feel around on the front wall. If you find an area that feels good to him, linger there. If not, hold your finger still or remove it for a short while as you focus on other forms of stimulation to bring the arousal up, then resume the search.

Try having him ejaculate while your fingers are inside him. You can feel the prostate swell dramatically just before he comes—if you were unsure of its location this will help you know where it is. And it's a nice way to round out the play session, since it feels damn good to rub the prostate during orgasm. Know that for most men, the ass tightens up right after ejaculation, so be sure to hold still for a moment after he comes, then pull out slowly.

8

BRINGING UP THE TOPIC: A GUIDE FOR HIM AND HER

WHY GUY–GIRL COUPLES ARE EXPLORING PROSTATE PLAY

More and more male–female pairs are discovering prostate play and having a grand time doing it. There are plenty of men who want to explore this, and who want to do it with a woman. Fortunately, there are lots of women who are happy to accommodate!

Why? To give him pleasure. Because it's hot to see him feeling so good. Because playing with taboo can be a real turn-on. For the excitement of trying something new. To do something "naughty." Because the role reversal of having her do the penetration while he receives it can be a thrilling new experience. And for the intimacy and trust that comes with him opening himself up in this way.

People who are interested in erotic dominance and submission may find that prostate play lends itself well because of the vulnerability involved and the possibility of a "forced" orgasm. Others may do it in a way that is totally vanilla, sweet and sensual, with no suggestion of dominance and submission.

Many straight couples simply view it as a natural turnabout for the attentions he may have given to her ass or G-spot. One couple learned about the "male G-spot" while looking for information about the female G-spot. The woman said, "We did research to stimulate mine and found information about his, and it piqued his curiosity." They had already played with her ass and explored her G-spot, so exploring his seemed like a perfectly natural next step.

THE BENEFITS OF TAKING TURNS

In addition to being lots of fun, prostate play can help improve your sex life in some surprising ways. First off, one of the more *"The bottoming I've done has really improved my topping."* common complaints of women about male partners is that they go too fast. A lot of guys want to rush right to the penetration, which can be difficult enough for vaginal sex, but it's especially likely to limit fun and pleasurable anal play. For most men, sex is something that happens outside the body. Once you've experienced what it's like to feel something enter your body, you're more able to realize how your mood, your emotions, and your physical sensations in that moment can affect your ability to catch instead of pitch. Not to mention that you develop a better appreciation for the value of warming up and getting turned on.

On the flip side, many women who use strap-on dildos discover how much work, responsibility, and (sometimes) power can be part of fucking someone. And they don't even need to worry about whether their penis will stay hard or ejaculate too soon! Lots of people we've spoken with have much more understanding and compassion for their partners after trying out prostate play, whether by hand or with toys. So when you try it out, pay attention to what you notice and what you feel. You just might find that the rest of your sex life gains a lot from the experience.

REASONS FOR HESITATION

Many men, especially straight men, are reluctant to tell their female partners that they want to explore prostate play. Sometimes it is the woman who wants to suggest this kind of play, but hesitates. If finding the prostate didn't involve going up his ass, it probably would not be so much of an issue—it would likely be viewed as no different from playing with any other part of the male sex equipment. But unfortunately, because our culture has a lot of baggage around the ass, anal pleasure, and male-receptive penetration in particular, all these issues come up for prostate play.

These concerns are common, but they are not impossible to overcome. If you or your partner has concerns about cleanliness, check out chapter 4, Hygiene. And if either of you has concerns such as "Who's playing the man's role?" or "Does it mean he's gay?," check out chapter 13, Real Men Don't, where we discuss these issues in depth.

> *"My partner was totally into it, and I actually started playing with his prostate and fucking him in the ass at his request. I did have some reservations about it (being from the Midwest and all); it truly was "the last taboo" for me, but his turn-on from it was undeniable and his desire was true, so I said yes, and was surprised at how much I enjoyed getting him off that way."*

> *"[...] I didn't raise the issue of anal play until after we had been having sex for a few months—I think out of concern that she might be repelled by the idea, but as it turned out she wasn't."*

> *"I think my boyfriend was shy about asking me to penetrate him because he had some shame and fear of rejection around his desire for anal play, but I had no inhibitions about it."*

> *"If it's something that he wants to try, and that I want to try, we'll do it."*

OPEN THE CONVERSATION

Bringing up the subject of prostate play can be a very easy thing or it can be rather complex. It depends a lot on your relationship with your partner, how they feel about prostate play and anal penetration, your sexual and relationship history together, and more. Fortunately, there are some pretty easy ways to introduce the topic.

If you have a trusted partner with whom you speak freely about sex, and you feel comfortable telling them directly about your new interest, by all means, do so! You could simply say, "I've been reading a lot about prostate massage, and I'm curious. Could we give it a go?" Or you could begin by asking what your partner knows about the prostate as a sex organ: "Have you heard of prostate massage?" If they don't know anything about it, you might need to bring them up to date before you ask if they are interested in trying it.

If this feels too risky to you, you can take a more subtle approach. You might open the conversation more casually: "I was web-surfing the other day and I found a website about prostate health. Did you know that prostate massage may benefit prostate health?" Just be mindful that sometimes this sneaky approach backfires! Some people are so conditioned to renounce "taboo" subjects of conversation that they would immediately deny any interest in prostate massage, because, ironically, they are afraid of what *you* might think of them if you thought *they* were interested.

Some men with female partners get into the conversation by talking about the prostate as the male equivalent of the G-spot—this works especially well if the couple has already been exploring her G-spot, or, for that matter, her ass. That way, she can relate to the pleasure that you are asking for. You might say, "Earlier today I read something about the 'male G-spot.' Have you heard of that?"

Whatever you do, don't say, "I've heard that some people— weirdos!—like to massage their prostate by sticking their fingers up their asses—of all places!—isn't that weird??" If you are going to feel out your partner's response by making a casual mention of the prostate, be sure to do it in a way that doesn't reinforce the stigma attached to male anal penetration. If you ask in a way that conveys ambivalence on your part, it isn't likely to dispose your partner to say yes.

For many people who have a freak-out response, it's not really about prostate massage—it's about male anal penetration. This is the real trigger, because this is what is loaded with taboo. To avoid this, deemphasize the idea of anal penetration and emphasize the prostate pleasure. Remind your partner that the prostate is actually a part of the male genital organs, but since it is buried deep in the pelvis, the way to reach it is through the neighboring rectum.

If you're hesitant to bring the topic up because you expect that your partner will have a negative reaction, you might want to reconsider. We've talked with people who held back from talking about prostate play and other kinds of sex only to discover that their partner was doing exactly the same thing! When you don't ask for what you want, you're a lot less likely to get it. If you talk about it, you still might not get it, but your odds improve a lot. So take a deep breath and ask what your partner thinks. They may also be trying to get up the courage to do just that.

Timing

When you are opening the conversation on a new and potentially touchy subject, timing is crucial. Make sure you have privacy—if your partner is tense about the subject, even people in the next room could put them on edge. Do it at a time when your partner is calm and relaxed and you are feeling open and connected.

Make sure that you are both available to talk at length if necessary. Don't do it before one of you has to rush off to a dinner date or a business meeting. Likewise, choose an opportunity when you can take some time to be apart if necessary, in case the conversation goes poorly.

It's often better to raise the topic when you're not having sex. That's because surprises during sex have an unfortunate tendency to trigger a bigger response, so if your partner has any negative reactions, they may get magnified. Of course, that's not always the case. Plenty of people have confessed their fantasies during the heat of passion and had it work out quite well. But lots of people have had the disclosure go awry because they brought it up during sex. We think your odds are better if you're not already turned on when you talk about it for the first time.

Lastly, if it's a new playmate, unless you have reason to think they'd be into this, it's probably a good idea to wait until you've had a few dates before you bring it up.

Ask with Confidence

When you do ask for it, ask with confidence. Whenever you are making any kind of pitch to anyone, your expectations have a major impact on the way you ask. And likewise, the way you ask has a big effect on the kind of answer you get.

If a fellow is expecting to be shot down, he might say, "So... I was kinda thinking that, you know, maybe...you could bend me over and...you know—use your hands on me. I mean—if you're into that!... Unless you don't want to..." Odds are, he will indeed get shot down! Your chances are much better if you give a confident delivery: "You know, I've heard a lot of good things about prostate massage. I know we've never done anything like that before but I'm curious to try. What do you think?"

Interest in prostate play is more common than most people realize. Even if your partner isn't interested in doing it with you, there's nothing wrong with you for wanting this. Remind yourself of that before you bring it up.

This may also open up a discussion about your partner's fantasies or desires. Make some room to hear about them and be as willing to explore them as you'd like your partner to be around your own interests. Who knows? This might be the start of a whole new phase in your erotic relationship.

BE FLEXIBLE

You never know how a person will react to being asked to explore prostate play. Be

"My wife feels that it's gross."

prepared for a variety of responses: they may be enthusiastic, they may be curious but hesitant, they may feel entirely neutral—not opposed, but not particularly jazzed either. They may be freaked out and completely against the idea. They may have several different feelings all at once. Try to be sensitive to their reaction.

If a freak-out happens, the initial reaction will tend to be the worst. Your partner may come around after talking with you about their concerns, but they may be too worked up to have that conversation right away, so give them a little space.

Don't bring it up again for a few days so they have time to think about it without feeling pressured.

When you reopen the conversation, you might ask directly: "What is it about the idea of prostate massage that bothers you?" Try to talk over their concerns without feeling defensive. If you think it would be helpful, give them this book to read. But don't push someone who simply isn't interested or try to shame them for being a prude—neither of these approaches will get you the enthusiastic playmate that you want.

A partner's lack of interest doesn't mean that there's something wrong with your desires. Whatever they are hung up on, it is about them—not about you. Preferences around sex are like preferences around food—just because your partner doesn't like cheesecake doesn't mean you shouldn't have a slice. Similarly, if your partner isn't interested in prostate play and you're monogamous, you can still have lots of fun with it on your own, using your fingers (if you can manage) or toys.

If you are in an ongoing relationship with a partner who is not interested in exploring your prostate with you, and you want to go it alone, we recommend that you be honest about this intention. If you hide it from them and they find out, they may be very hurt and upset. The act of hiding it sends the message *I'm doing something you think is wrong, so I need to keep it from you.* It will likely damage the trust in your relationship because they will wonder what else you might be keeping from them. It could easily turn out to be a bigger deal than it would have been if you'd been honest in the first place.

Sometimes all it takes to work things out is a little flexibility around how you'll do prostate play. For example, if your partner is OK with massaging your prostate with a finger but not strap-on play, or open to your wearing a butt plug during other kinds of sex, that gives you lots of options. And of course, maybe things will change over time, as they so often do. So rather than getting into a big fight over it, look for some common ground. This will be much easier if you can both be honest about your thoughts and feelings.

One of the most important things to remember when it comes to prostate play is that it can be incredibly fun for both the giver and the receiver. And something else to keep in mind: as with any kind of sex, it's not for everyone. So while we absolutely encourage you to introduce the topic, make room for your partner to have a different response. If they're not into it, suggest that they take a look at this book. Maybe the root of their reaction is unfamiliarity with the topic. And quite possibly, once they learn a bit about why people do it and how it works, they'll be up for giving it a shot too!

9

PROSTATE MASSAGE

WHAT IS PROSTATE MASSAGE?

The term *prostate massage* refers to the application of pressure to the prostate, with fingers or a toy, through the front wall of the rectum. It is also called "milking the prostate," since the massage often causes some prostatic fluid to be released and to run from the tip of the cock.

Because rubbing the prostate can feel like an entirely new kind of pleasure, it is often performed for purely erotic reasons. Some men say it feels like the first stage of an orgasm. This makes sense: the massage causes the prostate to swell and creates a feeling of compression, similar to what happens during ejaculation.

Prostate massage also has a long history of being performed

for medical purposes. Some believe that regular massage is beneficial to the health of your prostate. As with massage on many other parts of your body, it supports the natural processes of the organ, encourages circulation, removes any stuck fluids, and prompts the generation of new, fresh prostatic fluid. (For an in-depth discussion of the possible health benefits of prostate massage, see chapter 15.)

In this chapter, we focus on massage with fingers. Toys have their merits, but fingers have distinct advantages. Fingers are the most dexterous part of your body, so they offer an immense variety of sensation from the many different kinds of movement they can perform. You can feel the landscape in minute detail and you can touch with precision. Fingers can be added or subtracted at will, giving you many size options. And unlike toys, fingers give you a direct connection with your partner's body—fingertip to pleasure zone—which can feel deeply intimate.

Although it is possible for some men to massage their own prostate, these techniques work better with a partner, so that's who we'll be addressing. And if you haven't read chapter 7, Find It: Locating the Gland, we suggest starting there.

"Deliberate" Pressure

Many guides to prostate (and female G-spot) massage suggest that you apply "deliberate" pressure. What does that mean, exactly? It means that your fingers aren't flopping around like a fish in there. Rather, you are applying steady pressure in smooth, controlled strokes. Think of the motion you use to spread jam on toast: smooth and even. Even as you move in and out over the prostate, you're not just jabbing at random. Instead, you're maintaining contact as your finger slides across the surface and (for many techniques) keeping the level of pressure consistent across the whole surface. This is a kind of touch that many recipients will enjoy.

Poking versus Stroking

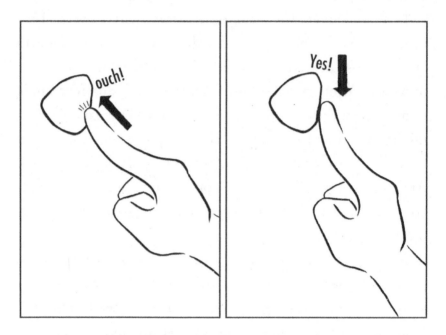

Illustration 7. Don't Poke It—Stroke It!

Here's a quick sensory experiment. Take your hand and place it on top of your opposite shoulder. Put two fingers together and press the fingertips into the meat of your shoulder. Now press using the pads of your fingers. Notice that even if you apply the same amount of pressure each time, the fingertips feel much more intense than the pads.

When you use the pads of your fingers, the pressure is distributed over a broader area, so the sensation feels more diffuse. In contrast, when using just the tips of your fingers, all the force is concentrated in a smaller area, creating a more intense poking sensation. To put it another way, pressure is force divided by area—for example, pounds per square inch. If the force stays the same, a greater area means less pressure.

When it comes to the prostate, poking is exactly what you don't want to do! It may have felt great on your shoulder just now, but the prostate is another matter entirely. We've spoken with a lot of men who complained about fingertips poking and stabbing their prostate, which can feel too intense, uncomfortable, or even painful. So be careful to avoid poking during the massage. Never drive directly into the gland with a motion like ringing a doorbell. Instead, apply moderate pressure using as much of your finger pads as possible to spread the sensation out. When you hold that pressure steady as you slide across the gland, you are effectively stroking, not poking.

Start Slow, Ramp Up

In the responses to our survey questions about prostate massage techniques, two words came up over and over again: *slow* and *gentle*. Most men can take, and enjoy, hard pressure and fast motion on the prostate during climax and during the states of high arousal leading up to it. But if you start the massage with that level of intensity, it's likely to feel overwhelming.

It's easy to fall into the trap of thinking that "more is better." Many people believe that harder and faster stimulation is the best way to create more sensation, but this is not always true. Think about spicy food. More intensity isn't always better—the best flavors come when the spices are balanced. Prostate massage is similar in that respect. When your partner isn't aroused enough to take the level of intensity that you are giving, it is likely to feel like too much.

If the stimulation continues to feel unpleasant, his nerves may reject the sensations by shutting off and numbing out, and then he definitely won't feel any pleasure. That, of course, is the opposite of the desired effect—so resist the temptation to go hard and fast right away. This is particularly important if he is new to prostate massage; he may be tender at first and going too hard may hurt. But even if he has experience, starting slow will serve you well.

At the start of each new massage, a little bit goes a long way, and seemingly mild touches can create decidedly intense sensations: it is all new to the body at that moment. To maximize the novelty factor at the start of each session, do slow strokes at the beginning. Easy does it! Since each tiny stroke feels so new to him, you might be surprised at how far you can take him along the road to pleasure with slow movements and fairly light pressure. Begin by applying only as much pressure as you'd use to check the ripeness of a piece of fruit.

As the energy builds, you can ramp up to higher levels of intensity in a way that works for him and will be enjoyable every step of the way. Throughout the session, build slowly from lower to higher levels of intensity. Every few minutes, increase the pressure a bit, or go a little faster.

To avoid going too far too quickly, follow a roller coaster model: increase the intensity for a spell, then drop it down a bit, then increase a little more, drop down, and so on. Each time you bring the intensity back down, you essentially press the Reset button on his nerves. Initially, the lighter sensations won't feel like much to him because of the harder stimulation of a moment before, but soon he will adjust to the lighter sensation and start picking up on it—then you can take him back as high as you were before, and even higher. Backing off and then heightening the intensity works for many different kinds of sex.

Rhythm and Variety

Rhythm is key to making any kind of sex play feel good, and prostate massage is no exception. Keeping a steady rhythm means you repeat whatever you are doing at consistent intervals for a given period of time without change.

When strokes are not repeated in a consistent rhythm, the motion can feel erratic and less pleasant. If you are constantly switching from fast to slow speeds and varying the motion of your stroke, your partner may find it difficult to relax into the sensation because he never knows what's coming. He may be just beginning to enjoy the slow little circles you are tracing over his prostate when suddenly they are interrupted by fast in-and-out strokes that are over as quickly as they began. If this goes on, he may find it difficult to enjoy himself.

A steady, repeated rhythm makes it much easier to get into

each sensation and enjoy it thoroughly. He can relax into the stroke and savor it. After all, what is easier to see: a single shooting star, or a meteor shower? This is why massage therapists frequently repeat a motion several times before moving on. Maintaining a steady rhythm is largely a matter of muscle memory, so it gets easier with practice.

If you can, try to rely on his responses to determine when it is time for a change. When he's really diggin' it, keep doing exactly what you're doing. As the authors of *Tantric Male Multiple G-spot Orgasm* point out, there's a common pitfall: you hear him getting really excited, so in your eagerness to please him, you intensify your strokes, abandoning the rhythm that you were using. "[I]t's only natural that you want to go faster and harder when you see and hear how great what you're doing is making him feel. But then you've changed what was working."[16]

Of course, eventually that little thing you do, having been repeated for a while, will start to lose its pizzazz. His body will get used to the touch and it won't feel so interesting anymore, so his response may become more moderate. Your hand may start to grow tired too. This is the time to switch to something different. When you introduce variety, you have many options. Here are the basic ones, which you can mix and match to get many more possibilities:

- Stroke—Switch it up! Go from in-and-out motion to circles, or side-to-side strokes. (We describe these strokes and many others later in this chapter.)

- Pressure—Lighten the pressure to ramp the energy

down or give your fingers a break. Increase the pressure when you want to take things back up again.

- Speed—Speed up or slow down to create fresh sensations. Or do a combination: fast-fast-slow, fast-fast-slow—repeating this set to create an interesting new rhythm.

- Location—Although the gland is fairly small, the prostate has different areas you can focus on. You might rub down the right lobe for several strokes, then move to the left lobe for several more. You can focus on the middle, the deep end, the lower half, or the gutters to either side. You will find that different parts of the prostate vary in sensitivity over time. One moment, rubbing the deep end of the prostate elicits an enthusiastic "Oh, right there!" But after 10–20 strokes, the deep end might yield less sensation, and rubbing the shallow end, which felt unremarkable to him before, suddenly drives him wild.

TIPS FOR COMBINING WITH COCK PLAY

For many men, prostate massage is the icing on the cake of tried-and-true oral sex or a hand job. Combining cock play with prostate massage has the benefit of broadening and unifying the sensations felt in the genitals, so he can sense the interconnection between all the genital parts, which we usually think of as being separate. However, for some men, simultaneous cock and prostate stimulation can be overwhelming simply because there's so much going on, especially if they are accustomed to focusing on just one part for pleasure.

If your partner is in this boat, start by alternating between cock and prostate and build slowly toward simultaneous stimulation of both. Have one hand on his cock and the fingers of the other on his prostate. As you stroke his cock, keep the fingers of your other hand inserted but hold them still. Then hold the hand on his cock still as you rub his prostate. There will be renewed excitement each time you switch (as you may notice from the moans) and you will be building the arousal of each part individually, so that eventually you can do both at once. And in the meantime, you are also getting the chance to practice each stroke on its own, so that your muscle memory will be better able to maintain these strokes smoothly when you are trying to do both in sync.

When you are ready, try both at once. This takes a certain amount of coordination and practice. It can be difficult to maintain a steady rhythm when doing two different motions to two different body parts, sort of like patting your head and rubbing your belly at the same time. But the more you practice, the easier it gets.

It's more important than ever to keep a steady rhythm now. Stimulating multiple erogenous zones at the same time can be hot, but if you do it in a sporadic, frenzied manner, it may just feel overwhelming or distracting. As you begin to move both hands at once, the thing to remember is this: rhythm is more important than speed!

Going slowly at first will make it easier for you to concentrate. Slow down as much as necessary to keep both hands moving at a steady rhythm. Don't worry if he loses his erection at this point. Reassure him that he doesn't need a hard-on for this to feel good. He will still enjoy the sensation of having his cock stroked, and chances are the erection will come back before too long.

Begin with both hands moving at the same tempo: one stroke on the prostate and one stroke on his shaft. As this becomes comfortable for him, you can increase the speed of both hands; you can also increase the tempo of one but not the other. Often the cock can take faster strokes than the prostate, so try staggering the rhythm: for example, one stroke on the prostate for every two strokes on the cock.

Reading Him

In an ideal world, you'd know exactly what he wants because *he'd* know exactly what he wants and he'd tell you. But often we don't know what we want, and even if we do, we don't always know how to ask for it. The best way to find out what he wants is to ask him. We recommend this as your first-line strategy. That being said, if you pay attention, you can also get a lot of information from his body language.

Is he undulating his hips rhythmically with your touch? That's probably good—keep doing what you're doing. Is he pressing his body toward you? Also good! This probably means he is begging for more intensity.

Sometimes it is hard to tell if squirming is a good sign or a bad one. If it is rhythmic, and if he is moving closer to you, it's usually a good sign. But if the movement is jerky and sudden, and if he is moving away from your touch, it may be a sign of discomfort.

One woman we spoke with told us about a time she played with a fellow who was jerking his hips around and moaning while she worked his prostate with her fingers. From the sound of it, she thought he was having a grand time. But in fact he was practically climbing up the headboard to move away from her. She asked him later about his squirming and he said that rather than writhing in pleasure, he had been trying to adjust the position of her hand, to give her cues as to where the right spot was—because she was missing it and uncomfortably applying pressure to another area of his ass. So gather whatever information you can from his body language, but when in doubt, ask!

HOW MANY FINGERS?

Preferences vary. Some are happy with just one, others prefer several. This depends largely on how tight his ass is and how big the fingers are.

One very slender finger may slip easily into a tight anus, but by virtue of being a single slender digit, it can easily deliver a sharp, poking sensation to the prostate. This is because one finger applies pressure to a smaller surface area, so the sensation will be very concentrated.

A thicker finger might be a little more difficult to insert into that same snug bottom, but it may feel better by virtue of delivering less of a poke. If you have skinny fingers, be very careful to use as broad a surface of your finger pad as possible and apply pressure evenly to the surface of the prostate. If the ass in question can accommodate more fingers, use more; this will broaden the sensation.

If you have shorter fingers, you may find that adding more fingers gives you more reach. Sometimes the lack of flexibility in your other fingers, which are being bent out of the way, can limit your ability to go deeper. Try this experiment: Holding your pinky and ring finger straight, bend your index finger and middle finger toward your palm. Do you feel tightness or tension in your hand? Now try it again, but just hold your pinky straight. Is that easier? What happens when you hold your index finger and pinky straight while bending your middle and ring fingers? A lot of people find that different combinations of fingers give them more movement and finesse, so see what works best for you. Also, the way you position the fingers that are not inside him will affect your reach.

If your hand starts to grow tired, change fingers to change which muscles you're working. Using different combinations of fingers also allows you to switch between techniques, so the workload is spread more equitably across your hand. If your thumb is long enough to reach the prostate, give it a try. It has more independent mobility than your fingers and allows for a number of positions that would not be comfortable for the other digits.

MASSAGE STROKES

The prostate responds pleasurably to a number of different strokes and motions. Here are several for you to try.

Side to Side

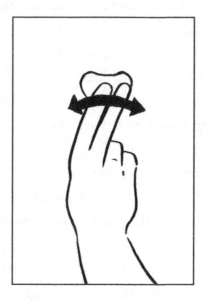

Illustration 8. Side to Side

Apply pressure to the prostate, holding the pressure as you slide over the surface from one side to the other and back. This stroke is sometimes called "windshield wipers."

In and Out

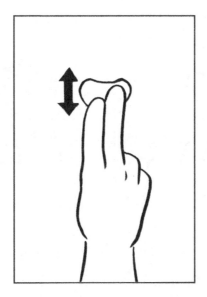

Illustration 9. In and Out

Reach your fingers in to the deep end of the prostate, apply pressure, and hold. Then drag your finger pads over the prostate from top to bottom. As you move back in, either release the pressure or maintain it, as long as you are very careful not to poke inward.

Circles

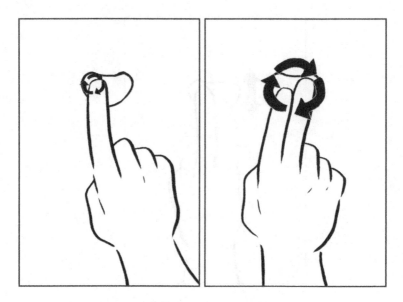

Illustration 10. Circles

Apply and maintain constant pressure as you slide over the surface of the gland, tracing a circle. You can trace small, localized circles so that only your fingers move, or cover the whole surface of the gland: north, east, south, and west. Be sure to try both clockwise and counterclockwise motion.

Come-Hither

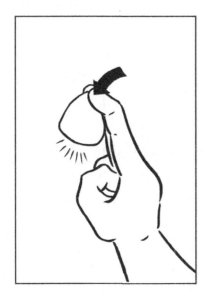

Illustration 11. Come-Hither Curl

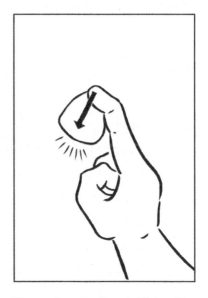

Illustration 12. Come-Hither Tug

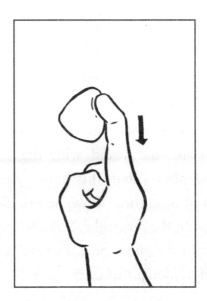

Illustration 13. Come-Hither Slide

This stroke is the most evocative of the phrase "milking the prostate" because when you use this stroke, you pump the gland downward, moving the fluids in their natural direction toward the prostatic urethra. Place your fingertips on the deep end of the prostate, as far as you can reach, so that the gentle curve of your fingers nestles against the rounded top of the gland. At this point, you have a few options.

1) Keep your hand stationary and curl your fingers as if you were gesturing "come here." Continue pressing and releasing. Since only your fingers move in this position, it is well suited for tight asses that aren't up for much in-and-out motion. We call this the "Come-Hither Curl."

2) Keep your fingers in the curled position, and move your entire hand slightly in and out, maintaining contact with the deep end of the prostate at all times and gently tugging at it with an inward, downward motion toward the cock. This is the "Come-Hither Tug."

3) In the "Come-Hither Slide," you slide your fingers out, just as you would with the In and Out, described above, but this time, you curl your fingers and drag them down across the surface of the gland on the outstroke. Straighten your fingers on the instroke and repeat. Be sure your nails are short before doing this one!

Vibration

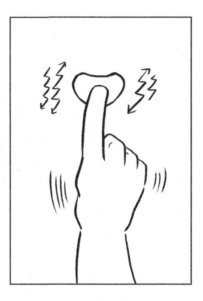

Illustration 14. Vibration

Apply pressure to the prostate and hold the pressure without any motion. Then, maintaining the pressure, use very small, very rapid motions of your hand from side to side, creating vibration. For this stroke, you barely move from the original position—it is a very localized motion. Vibration combines nicely with other strokes: for example, instead of vibrating in just one location, continue vibrating as you trace your fingertips in a circle over the whole gland. You can add vibration to any other stroke by doing both simultaneously. Or, take advantage of technology: make any stroke vibrate by holding a vibrator against the palm of your hand during penetration.

Jostling

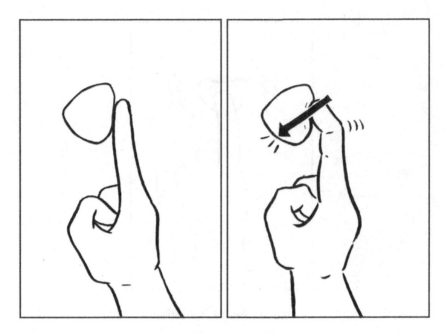

Illustration 15. Jostling

Jostling is like vibration in that you are maintaining constant contact with the prostate, but instead of doing small, rapid motions, you bounce the prostate on your fingertips, jostling it.

Tapping

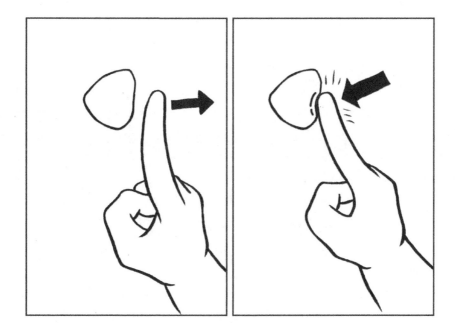

Illustration 16. Tapping

With a small, quick motion, lift your finger off the prostate and let it drop back down again, percussing the prostate as you would type on a keyboard. This is a very small motion but can create a powerful and pleasant sensation. You can do this with one finger, or several fingers held together. A variation, if you have two or more fingers inserted, is to wiggle your fingers separately, like spider's legs, so that they strike the prostate alternately.

Twisting

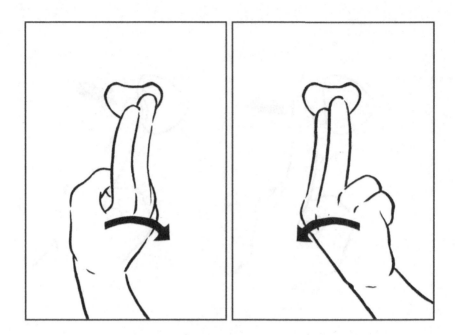

Illustration 17. Twisting

With your finger inserted, apply pressure and repeatedly rotate your hand at the wrist, so that your finger twists clockwise, then counterclockwise. This will be more compelling with two or more fingers so there is broader area on the prostate where the twisting motion can be felt.

Scissors

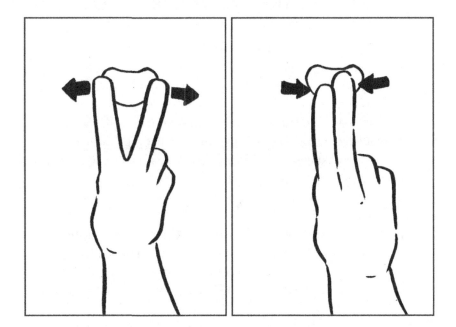

Illustration 18. Scissors

Rest two fingers on the midline of the gland, between the two lobes. Then, maintaining a constant pressure on the gland, spread your fingers apart, and with the same even pressure, close them again. You can also do this on each lobe. This stroke may be difficult if the receiver has a very tight anus. Sex educator Robert Morgan Lawrence has a handy tip for this: increase your finger strength by practicing with a rubber band!

TAKE CARE OF YOUR BODY

As you give a prostate massage, pay attention to the needs of your body. How does your wrist feel? Your back? This goes for both partners: you can play longer if you are gentle with yourselves so that you aren't putting strain on your joints or becoming sore.

To increase endurance, vary the part of your body that you use to create the motion. For example, imagine that your partner is on his hands and knees in front of you, and you are kneeling behind him. Your fingers are on his prostate (with your palm facing down, of course), and you are doing an in-and-out stroke. You can do this stroke moving only from the wrist. With your finger pads on his prostate, simply bend your wrist backward on the outstroke, so that your knuckles rise toward the ceiling, and unbend it again on the instroke. This motion gets the job done, but it puts all the work on your wrist, which will tire quickly and may even begin to feel sore and strained.

However, in this same position, you can use other muscles and other joints to create the motion and give your wrist and hand a break. Keeping your wrist and finger joints at the same angle, move in and out by swinging your whole arm very slightly forward and backward from the shoulder joint. To give your shoulder a break, keep your whole arm *and* shoulder stationary, and simply rock your torso forward and backward.

To keep your wrists in good shape, do a few mild stretches before each session.

FISTING

"How many fingers do you or your partner(s) like to insert for P-spot stimulation?"

"All of them."

Anal fisting is the practice of inserting into the anus all five fingers and, while you're at it, the whole hand down to the wrist or deeper. You start with a couple of fingers, and if it feels good, you add a couple more. And if that still feels good, you tuck the thumb alongside them, forming the "duck's bill." And, very gradually, given a very relaxed bottom, a very patient top, and generous amounts of lube, the whole hand can slide in down to the wrist.

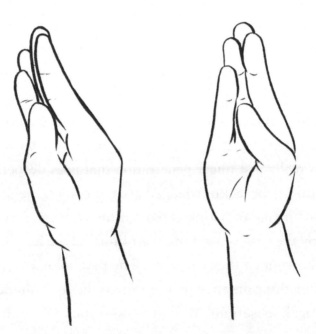

Illustration 19. The Duck's Bill: Hand Position for Fisting Penetration

A hand is often larger than the average butt toy (but not all!), so fisting is generally the domain of more experienced players. With increased size comes a greater risk of injury, so a significant amount of care and skill is required.

Some people find the idea of fisting alarming. This is likely due to the intimidating size of a fist. Since many people already have the expectation that being penetrated will hurt, the idea of being penetrated with something of considerable size makes it seem that much scarier. In addition, it doesn't help that the term *fisting* has as its root the word *fist*, which brings up violent associations such as punching someone. The word also suggests that you insert the whole closed fist into the anus all at once.

Of course that's an alarming image. It's also not how most people do fisting. As described above, it's preferably done slowly and gently, with a gradual transition from fewer to more fingers. You only close your fingers into a fist, if desired, once you are fully inside. Most fisters keep their fingers extended.

As long as entry isn't forced, anal fisting can be done more or less safely. In fact, doctors occasionally insert a whole hand into a patient's rectum for a medical procedure after dilation. Fisting is really just finger penetration that goes deeper.

It needs to be acknowledged that for some people, the "extreme" image of fisting is part of the turn-on. Recipients may enjoy the rush of pushing their limits to see how far they can go, how much they can take. The psychological thrill of doing something intense or taboo may be an enhancer for the physical sensation: "Oh my god—your whole hand is inside me!"

But for many people who get into fisting, it can be just like any other kind of sex play. It can be sensual and loving. Because of the vulnerability of opening yourself up in this way, it can inspire deep feelings of trust between partners. And because it can take a great deal of time and relaxation to open enough to accommodate your partner's hand, it can feel meditative and even ritualistic.

Also, if you take your time and build to the point where you can open to all the sensations that are coming your way, fisting can be quite a field day for the nerves of the anus, rectum, and prostate! Fisting can be incredibly stimulating to the prostate: when you have your whole ass filled up, there is more pressure in every direction, so it is much easier to apply pressure to the extra-sensitive places.

Fisting and Safety
While many people are able to do fisting relatively safely, it is important to acknowledge the risk involved. If you're new to fisting and are interested in exploring this erotic avenue, we highly recommend doing further research to be sure that you are doing it safely. We're covering the basics to give you a starting point, but you should know that there's a lot more to be said on the topic. See the Resources for some useful guides.

When it comes to fisting, many people have the ambition but lack the physical ability. We'd like to reiterate the importance of listening to your body. You could seriously hurt yourself if you aren't careful. If you choose to use alcohol or other substances while being fisted, make absolutely sure that you are sober enough to feel any pain that might arise and you are able to stop doing whatever is causing it.

When you penetrate someone with a very large object—or do any penetration roughly and carelessly—it is possible to perforate the rectum, which means a trip to the emergency room. It's probably not a problem if you notice a small amount of faintly pinkish tinge to the lube when you wipe up after fisting—this can occasionally happen during anal penetration. However, if the fistee is actually bleeding red blood during or after being fisted, they should go to the hospital. Also, if they have a fever on the following day, they should seek immediate medical attention, as this may be a sign of perforated colon.

"Before anyone starts I need to have a trust/comfort/feeling that the person who will fist me will look out for my well-being and be caring. [...] I have had more failures than successes, where after 3–4 fingers I know this is not going to work, and once my comfort is gone then it's just not going to happen."

An enema is highly recommended before fisting. Fecal matter can be abrasive and make penetration by such a large object uncomfortable. (See chapter 4, Hygiene, for enema tips.) Also, be extra generous with lube! Lubricants that are popular for fisting include vegetable shortening and J-lube. (See chapter 11, Toys, for more information on lube.)

Before you begin, the fister should remove any rings and make sure that their fingernails are filed short and smooth. Gloves are a good idea, not only to protect the hand and any small cuts on the hand from body fluids, but also to smooth out the hand and minimize discomfort for the fistee. Make sure the gloves fit snugly—bunchy gloves won't feel nearly so nice!

Most disposable gloves are not very long, but the prostate isn't very deep, so you can usually get by with these. In most cases, they are just long enough to cover the whole hand and wrist. However, it's possible for lube to drip from the glove onto your wrist, depending on your position. This is unlikely to be a problem as long as the skin is unbroken. Just be sure to wash the area thoroughly with soap and water afterward to keep things clean.

If the prostate is only a stop on the way and you plan to explore deeper penetration, consider getting longer gloves. There are a number of options for this, though they tend to be more expensive than your average-size disposable gloves. Consult online medical and dental suppliers to find extra-long disposable gloves (12 inches instead of the usual 9 inches).

A number of online BDSM toy retailers carry latex or rubber gloves that are elbow length or longer, including some that fit over the whole hand, binding the fingers snugly together in a duck-bill-like position. These gloves are somewhat porous, so there's no guarantee of getting them 100 percent clean. Some people wash them and reuse them with the same partner, but it's important to know that they've never been tested for safety the way surgical gloves are. They wear out after three to seven uses, depending on the brand. So if you like how they look and feel, remember that they can be hard to keep clean and they'll wear out.

Insertion Technique

Opening the ass to a fist is all about relaxation. Not everyone has the ability to relax as fully as necessary to do this safely. You may not be able to accommodate a whole fist on your first attempt. Some people never will. We appreciate that taking a whole fist is a hot fantasy for many people, but try not to maintain the goal of getting the whole thing inside, and never force penetration. It should feel good during the entire experience—not just after you "go all the way."

Be sure to set aside plenty of time. Open your partner slowly, working your way from fewer to more fingers, or smaller to larger toys. Use lots of lube and reapply often. When you have four fingers in, you can tuck your thumb alongside your fingers and gently press in.

Try pressing a little, then withdrawing a little, repeating in this fashion as you make your way in. You can also try gently twisting your hand. Feel your way in carefully: once your fingers are through the sphincters, you will have to gently navigate the soft folds of the rectum, which curve in a slightly different pattern on every person. Once the hand is inserted and the sphincters settle around the wrist, you can slowly, one finger at a time, draw your fingers in toward your palm to close your hand into a fist. This is not necessary, but it's a convenient hand position for many of the techniques described below.

Massaging the Prostate While Fisting

With your fist inserted, you may find that very subtle movements are enough to send your partner into prostate heaven.

It is also very easy to overstimulate the gland while fisting, so be sure to alternate between prostate-focused motions and holding still or moving in a way that applies less focused pressure on this area. Here are some techniques for massaging the prostate while fisting:

With your partner lying on his back and your hand inside him, close your fingers into a fist. Position your hand as if you were going to give someone a "thumbs up"—but don't actually lift your thumb, just let it sit flat on top of the closed fist. This positions the back of your thumb against his prostate. Now there are several ways you can pleasure his prostate with subtle motions of the thumb.

1. You can bend the thumb knuckle, causing the back of the thumb to lift into the prostate, and flatten again, repeatedly. Do this right down the midline of the prostate, or focus on one lobe for several strokes and then move to the other.

2. You can swivel the thumb right to left, mimicking the "windshield wiper" side-to-side massage technique.

3. Put the two together by lifting the back of the thumb up against the prostate, moving from right to left across the prostate, then flattening the thumb and moving from left to right to return to the original position; repeat. After several strokes, do it in the opposite direction so you press into the prostate on the left-to-right stroke. This is a fairly small motion—it doesn't take much!

4. As an alternative to technique #1 above, instead of moving the thumb, hold it still against the closed fist and pivot the whole fist up and down, moving from the wrist, so that the back of the thumb presses into the prostate.

5. With the thumb in the same position, hold it still against the closed fist and swivel your whole hand clockwise and counterclockwise in a twisting motion. You can do this with the thumb against the prostate (as an alternative to #2), or rotate your hand so that the punching knuckles of the index and middle finger dance over the prostate.

6. Keeping your fist closed, gently move the whole fist in a subtle in-and-out motion. (Not all the way in and all the way out—just a few centimeters so you rub up and down against the prostate.)

With fisting, a little goes a long way, so keep your motions small and slow. Don't make any fast moves—and that includes when you are pulling out at the end of play. If pain arises for your partner, hold still and have him breathe and relax until it passes. If it doesn't go away, remove your hand very slowly. Avoid the temptation to pull out quickly, even if your partner asks you to, because you could damage the tissue by doing so.

10

THE "SWEET SPOT": MASSAGING THE PERINEUM

Behind your balls, in front of your asshole, and squarely between your legs is the perineum. This unassuming (and often ignored) part of your body has a lot of erotic potential. Many people enjoy light caresses, licking, gentle touch, and vibration on the surface of the perineum. But that's not all. The prostate is just a couple of inches inside the perineum. It's close enough to the surface that if deep, focused touch is applied at the right spot, the pressure is transferred through the intermediate tissue and can be felt in the prostate. The sensations will feel less focused, sort of like rubbing some-one's shoulders through a sweater rather than massaging on bare skin, but that certainly doesn't mean it won't feel good!

Some have called this "the sweet spot." You might not

find pressing the spot to be much fun on its own. However, this external spot combines quite nicely with other kinds of play, such as hand jobs and blow jobs. It adds an extra zip, broadening the focus of stimulation so you can reach higher levels of arousal. Many will find that their orgasms feel more powerful if this point is pressed during climax. Plus, if you are curious about your prostate but not quite ready to go the anal route, this is a convenient way to dip your toes in the water.

Perineum massage is also a great way to intensify a prostate massage via the anal route. By applying pressure through the basement and the back door simultaneously, you are coming at the prostate from multiple angles. If you are warmed up enough to take this level of intensity, it can double the pleasure.

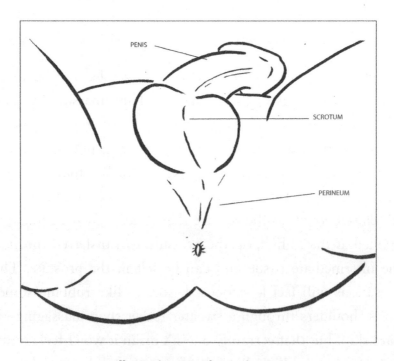

Illustration 20. The Perineum

WHY THE SWEET SPOT FEELS GOOD

If you flip back to chapter 3 and review Illustration 1, Male Anatomy, you can see that the bulb of the penis runs well into the body, extending partway into the perineum. Perched atop and slightly behind it is the prostate. It's fairly close to the surface, so when you massage the perineum with deep pressure in the right spot, that pressure is transmitted through to the prostate.

Some people feel prostate sensations when they press through the bulb of the erect penis. Others feel these sensations when they press into the soft area behind the bulb of the penis. The location of the spot is a little different for everyone, but it is generally along the midline between your legs.

As a bonus, in addition to being able to massage the prostate through the perineum, you can also massage the bulb of the cock. This deep end of your cock, which probably gets very little attention by comparison with the rest of the shaft, will appreciate the attention. This not only feels good but can also pump up your erection by pushing the blood through the blood vessels and further into the cock.

Some men report that when they reach the right spot, they feel a tingling sensation that radiates through their penis, perineum, prostate, and anus simultaneously. This makes the sensation feel more broad. It's not just your cock where you feel pleasure, but your cock in connection to the perineum, prostate, and anus.

On top of all that, when you massage the perineum, you can help the muscles of the pelvic floor relax. This increases blood flow, which is important for both sexual health and arousal. And if you're new to anal play, you may discover that it can also make penetration easier. When the muscles around the anus are tight, the anus is also likely to be tight, so massage can help relax the muscles and make penetration more comfortable.

FINDING THE SWEET SPOT

Since the prostate is a couple of inches inside the body, you need to use deep tissue massage to stimulate it through the perineum. Light touches only stimulate the surface nerves of the skin, as when you run your fingertips across the head of your cock. This can feel great, and will certainly be a nice way to "warm up" the area and build arousal. But it's not going to be felt in the prostate because it doesn't go deep enough. You need to apply firm, deep pressure to transfer the sensation to the prostate through the intermediate tissue.

Also, like so many things sexual, this is most likely to feel good if you are already turned on. Arousal makes the whole genital area more engorged and sensitive, so that when you apply pressure it is more likely to feel good. If you are unaroused, you might only feel pressure without any kind of erotic charge, or even discomfort. So before you get started trying to massage the prostate through your perineum, get yourself excited. Whether that means stroking your cock, fantasizing, massaging the anal opening, or anything else, get the blood moving before experimenting with your sweet spot.

If you are new to prostate sensations, what you feel may be

very subtle at first, even if you are turned on and pressing in the right area. Because this is an indirect massage, for many people it may take some practice to feel it in the prostate. As with many new things, it may not happen right away. If you try it a few times, you may discover new sensations.

FIND YOUR OWN

To find your sweet spot, you need to reach down between your legs, either from the front or from behind. If you're reaching from the front, make your back round to bring your perineum closer to your head. For example, lie down with a pillow under your head and another under your hips. Bring your knees up toward your face and reach your hand between your legs from the front. Or sit on a chair with your legs up on a table and reach between your legs from the front. You can also squat and reach down, though you may find this position difficult on your knees. Kneeling and rounding your back also works well.

If you want to reach from behind, arch your back. You can lie on your side with your top leg bent and resting on a pillow for easy access. Or get on your hands and knees and use one hand to reach back. If you can't support your weight on one hand, rest your torso on a chair or bed with your knees or feet on the floor.

Start Looking

As mentioned above, you are most likely to get a kick out of pressing your sweet spot if you are already excited. Once you are turned on and in a comfortable position, you are ready to start looking. If your cock is erect, find the rounded ridge that runs along the underside. This is the corpus spongiosum—one of the three erectile columns that run the length of the cock. Follow the ridge down the shaft and past your balls. It continues all the way into the perineum. You might even be able to feel where the root of the penis splits. This is where the corpora cavernosa—the other two cylinders that form the shaft of the cock—spread in a Y shape.

Place the tips of one or two fingers directly behind the scrotum and push in, holding for several seconds before releasing. Then move your fingers about a quarter inch further backward (away from the balls, toward the asshole), and repeat the press-and-release. Continue this at quarter-inch increments until you reach the hole, then start over from the scrotum. Experiment with different degrees of pressure, but don't go harder than is comfortable. For most men, the location of the sweet spot is much closer to the anus than the balls, but it's a little different for everyone.

Hopefully, as you do this perineum massage exercise, you'll find an area where the pressure feels a little different. It may be subtle at first, almost like a slight tingle. With a little practice, you'll be able to identify the sensation more easily and it can feel much stronger and more pleasurable. When you find a spot that feels different, stop and linger there. Massage it with deep, long presses, holding for several seconds, then releasing for several seconds. As you get used to the sensation, you can try a more rapid pulsation. Or dig in and hold the pressure while vibrating your fingertip with very small, quick back–and–forth motions. Press in and move your finger in a small circle. Just be careful not to dig in with your fingernails.

Don't forget to keep breathing. If you're holding your breath, you're probably also tightening your pelvic floor, which cuts down on the sensation and makes things harder to feel. If you've stopped touching your penis, go back to it and see how it feels to do both at the same time. Keeping the arousal up will make it easier to find the sweet spot.

If you massage the sweet spot during orgasm, you may feel the bulb of the penis swell with each contraction. Your ejaculation might not come out with as much force, since you're pressing on the tube that semen comes through, but it can often feel more intense.

Sit on It

Some men simply aren't built to comfortably reach their own sweet spot. If you have trouble reaching it with your fingers, and you don't have an available partner to do it for you, there are lots of objects you can use to massage your perineum. Some men sit on a rolled-up sock or a tennis ball while jerking off in order to apply pressure to the perineum. Try sitting on it and rocking back and forth or side to side to work it deep into the perineum.

One company even manufactures a toy for exactly this purpose: the Prostate Cradle is an external prostate massager made of silicone and shaped like a narrow bicycle seat. It's designed so you can sit on it and massage the sweet spot. It's worth noting, however, that the prostate cradle is marketed primarily as a health product, and the manufacturer takes a slightly squeamish approach to prostate massage via anal penetration, which it describes as "invasive." Because you're reading this book, we're guessing that you're more open to the idea of anal play—perhaps even enthusiastic about it—but if you want to try the prostate cradle, don't let this anal phobia stop you.

For a little extra zip, use a vibrator. In addition to applying pressure, a vibrator transmits sensation deep into the perineum. Some men are skeptical or uncomfortable about the suggestion that a vibrator might feel good for them: since vibrators are popular among women, there is a widespread assumption that they are only for women.

However, many men have tried applying vibration to their sensitive parts and found that it feels good. After all, in spite of differences in the structure of male and female genitals, the different organs respond in similar ways. The nerve endings like what they like, and it's just as simple as that! If you have a vibrator handy, give it a shot and see for yourself. (While you're at it, try pressing the vibe against the head of your cock!)

If you're using one of the long, skinny vibrators, you can massage the sweet spot with the tip. However, please note that many battery vibrators are not safe for anal penetration. If your toy doesn't have a base, please don't insert it—it can slip all the way inside and not come back out. That can mean going to the emergency room, so play it safe and only use toys with a base for anal penetration.

PARTNER MASSAGE

Having a partner massage your sweet spot can simplify matters considerably. In many positions, your partner can reach your perineum much more comfortably than you can—which lets you experience the massage in a way that is relaxed and free of wrist strain. As long as your partner is in a comfortable position, they can probably do it longer than you could by yourself. Plus, having your partner explore this sensitive zone may make it feel that much more fun.

Of course, you lose the direct biofeedback that you have with self-stimulation because your partner can't feel what you are feeling—only you can. So you might have to give them some guidance: "Higher. Lower. Not so hard... A little to the left. More pressure—good spot! Stay there!" Sometimes it might be a simple "I don't feel anything, but keep trying." Guiding your partner is much easier if you have already found your sweet spot by yourself: you will have some idea of the sensation that you are trying to spark.

A Guide for Partners

Before you start using deep pressure to look for the sweet spot, get your partner warmed up with light touches. Rub your fingers softly across the skin, with or without a lubricant, or run your tongue up and down the area while going down on him. Try with both hard and soft tongue. (A hard tongue is flexed and pointy, whereas a soft tongue is relaxed and soft, as if you were licking an ice cream cone.)

When he is ready, you can begin to apply a deeper pressure. One of you can rub his cock or stimulate other parts of his body at the same time to help eroticize the new sensations. Start with a broad massage of the perineum: close your hand into a ball and press the flat surface of your fingers into the perineum, or press in with the knuckles. Try this in a wave motion: roll your fist over the perineum as if you were kneading bread dough, applying pressure in a wave across the whole perineum.

Now you might begin the search for the sweet spot with more focused, deep pressure. You can use the tips of one or more fingers, or your thumb. Try vibration, pressing in with a finger or two while moving your hand back and forth in very small, rapid motions. Try pulsations, pressing, and releasing at various speeds. Somraj Pokras and Jeffre TallTrees, authors of *Tantric Male Multiple G-spot Orgasm*, suggest that this feels particularly good because it replicates the way the prostate contracts rhythmically during ejaculation.

If you have a finger or two massaging his prostate from the inside, use the thumb of that hand or your other hand to press into the sweet spot. Better yet, if your fingers and thumb are long enough, you can insert fingers and use the thumb to press into the prostate, or vice versa.

Listen to his feedback and follow the signs of his body. Ask him to tell you if you push too hard and it feels painful or uncomfortable.

If he wants to ejaculate, try pressing into the sweet spot during ejaculation. You can press and hold, or try a rapid press-and-release pulsation that mimics the contractions that occur during orgasm.

"I DON'T FEEL ANYTHING"

It may take a while to feel the sweet spot, during this session or over the course of several sessions, so don't give up right away. Have fun doing whatever you normally do, and let this exploration be the icing on the cake. Be sure to keep up familiar forms of stimulation so that the arousal stays high.

If you are pressing all over the perineum and can't find anything, give it a break. Do some other kind of sex play and try again in five minutes. If you're not sure you're in the right spot, try it during ejaculation. This will maximize your ability to feel the spot, since the prostate is swollen at this point and more sensitive to pressure. If you don't find it today, you can always try again another time. Keep practicing by yourself during masturbation, and remember that this is all about feeling good.

11

TOYS

LUBE

When it comes to making sex feel better and work better, there's nothing more effective than lubricant. Working the prostate without lube is like going down a water slide without running water. It's not nearly as fun, and it's likely to hurt!

The inside of your ass does not produce lubrication the way a vagina can. It comes equipped with only a thin layer of mucus that lines and protects the tissue. That lining is disrupted very quickly if you don't use lube, and the friction of a cock or anal toy rubbing against your delicate internal tissue may cause small, painful tears, irritation, and a sore bottom tomorrow.

Could you get by without it? Say, if you were just doing a

quick two-finger massage? Well, it's certainly been done. But why would you want to? Lube feels really, really good! Just as a back massage is better with massage oil, using lube during prostate massage will create a slickety-smooth and luxurious feeling. It also allows playtime to last longer because you won't get worn out so quickly, and that may help you reach higher levels of arousal and pleasure.

Lube is available in a wide spectrum of prices suited for every budget. Sex shops and Internet merchants catering to the adult market have the most impressive array of options, but these days many drugstores carry several options as well.

The kind of lube you want depends on the kind of play you are doing. If there is minimal motion, as with wearing a butt plug or getting a brief finger massage, you may get by just fine on that drugstore-brand lube. However, for activities that involve more motion, such as fucking, or larger objects, or for long-duration play sessions, you'll get the best performance from a lube that was made with these activities in mind.

Water-Based Lube

Water-based lubricants are a lube of convenience: they are widely available in a variety of textures, can be used with any kind of toy or safer sex barrier, and rinse off easily when you are finished. Plus, they're usually less expensive than other versions.

Some back door enthusiasts complain that water-based lubes dry out too quickly. This is particularly true of the thin, runny varieties. These feel great going in the ass—slippery, wet, and cooling—but the feeling doesn't last long because the water portion of the lube quickly evaporates or gets absorbed by the rectal tissue. That is, after all, part of what the lower colon does: absorb water back into the body.

By comparison, thicker water-based lubricants last much longer in the ass, and are favored by many prostate players. These lubes often have a gel-like consistency, which allows them to form a cushiony protective coating over the rectal lining, reducing friction more effectively than their thinner cousins.

Of course, whether it's thick or thin, when a water-based lube dries out, that sticky residue is lube-minus-water, so a little bit of water or spit can return it to its former slippery grandeur—sometimes more effectively than applying another dab of lube.

Glycerin is a common ingredient in water-based lubes. If a lube contains glycerin, it tends to get sticky when it dries out. Glycerin-free lubricants don't dry out, but they soak in like hand cream, so you may have to apply more of it. Some people find glycerin-based lube irritating when they use it for anal penetration. If you experience irritation, discomfort, or a burning sensation after playing with a glycerin-based lube, try a glycerin-free variety next time and see if it makes a difference.

J-LUBE

If you are doing extensive sessions of anal penetration, try J-lube. It is manufactured as a lube for veterinarians to use on animals during gynecological exams and insemination, but it has been adopted as the lube of choice of many anal players, especially for extensive sessions, large objects, and fisting.

It comes as a powder that you mix with water to create the desired amount of lube. A little bit goes a long way: 8 ounces of the powder can make—no joke—up to 8 *gallons* of lube, so it'll last a long time. You can use more water to make a thinner lube, or less to make a thicker lube. Needless to say, it will be more space efficient if you don't mix more than you need. Type "J-Lube" into your search engine and you'll find several online retailers.

Silicone

Silicone-based lubricants feel slick and almost oily, but unlike oils, they are latex safe. And unlike water-based lubes, they do not rinse off with water, which makes them ideal for playing in the shower, but also means that clean up is a bit more involved. Even after scrubbing thoroughly with soap, you might still feel a thin residue on your skin. And if you spill some on the floor, be sure to wipe it all up or you might slip on it, even hours or days later.

There's a chance that you're already using silicone products in your shaving cream, because they give you a slick, smooth shave. If dimethicone, dimethiconol, or cyclomethicone is in the ingredient list, it's the stuff in some of the common silicone lubricants.

They tend to be more expensive than water-based lubes, but you'll probably use a smaller amount, so they can be cost-effective despite the higher price for the same size bottle. Some silicone lubes may damage some silicone toys, so put a condom over the toy to keep it working right.

Many people rave about silicone lubricants because they never seem to dry out. The more slippery ones aren't ideally suited for lots of motion because the slick feeling they create is very different from the slippery wet feeling of a water-based lube.

If you are doing minimal motion, such as a finger massage or using a small toy, a silicone lube will do just fine, even if it is on the runnier side. However, a thicker variety protects the tissues better and is more suitable for play that involves larger objects or more movement, such as a fucking motion with a dildo.

MIX AND MATCH

You can have the best of both, or several, worlds by mixing various lubes together. Some people like to start anal penetration with a viscous lube such as a thick silicone or a gel-like water-based lube. This forms a base coat that will resist drying and will cling to the tissue, protecting against friction. Then, in order to allow for rapid motion, a thinner, wetter lube may be applied on top. You can switch back and forth between your lube bottles throughout play as you please. Or you can mix a water-based and a silicone lube together in a third bottle. This ensures that the proportions are always the same, although you'll need to experiment to find the combination that you like best. If they separate out, just give the bottle a shake before getting started.

Oil-Based Lube

Perhaps you've heard of a certain brand of vegetable short-ening that is an old favorite in some anal play circles? Very few of the products that are marketed and sold as sex lubes are oil based, but quite a few common oil-based household products have been adopted by prostate enthusiasts as a lube of choice. Vegetable shortening, coconut oil, and Albolene-brand moisturizer were not made to be used for sex, but plenty of men use them with no complaints. They feel super slick and are very long lasting. The creamy, semisolid vari-eties, like vegetable shortening, heat up to body temperature, which makes them take nicely to motion while still coating the rectum thoroughly.

On the downside, oil breaks down latex very quickly, which means that you shouldn't use oil with latex condoms or gloves. Nonlatex gloves and condoms are widely available for people with latex allergies, and these can be used with oil. (See chapter 4, Hygiene, for information on nonlatex barriers.)

If you do choose an oil, avoid anything with perfume in it like some massage oils or baby oils, as this may irritate the sensitive skin of the anus and rectum. Also, mineral oils like Vaseline or baby oil can actually dry tissues out, so go with a vegetable oil. Store the oil in the refrigerator to keep it from going rancid and pour some into a bowl when you want to play, to avoid contaminating the container. Coconut oil and almond oil are very popular choices, or you can buy one designed for sex.

TOY TIPS

So you want to buy a toy for your prostate? Excellent! Toys are a great way of stimulating the P-spot, with or without a partner. Sex toys offer unique textures and sensations, in addition to the thrill of novelty. They allow for ease of position and extended reach, as many men cannot comfortably stimulate their own prostate with their hands for a long period of time. A wide range of toys can be used to get to the P-spot, as long as you follow a few simple safety guidelines.

Anything you put into the anus should be smooth. Lots of toys have bumps or ridges for vaginal stimulation, but the anus is much more sensitive. To avoid pain, go for something smooth. Subtle, rounded ridges are OK and can feel really good, especially as they slide down over the prostate on the outstroke—just be mindful that it'll make for a bumpy ride, so go a little slower.

Make sure that your toy has a flared base. When you're shaking all over and your muscles are contracting and everything is slippery, a toy without a flared base can accidentally get pushed all the way into the ass too deep for you to pull it out. This has happened to plenty of people—so as tempting as that candle or cucumber may be, it's probably not worth the risk of a very uncomfortable trip to the emergency room.

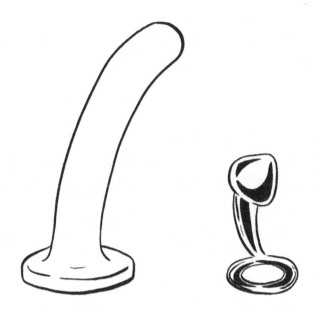

Illustration 21. Toys with Flared Bases

If you do lose a toy inside you, don't panic. Try taking a slow breath and see if you can push it out on the exhale. If that doesn't work, take a warm bath to help the muscles relax, and it might be easier to remove it. Some people report that drinking warm tea or eating something spicy stimulates the contractions of the digestive system and helps push the toy out. If these tips don't work, get to the emergency room. It's possible to damage the rectum or the colon, causing serious problems. As embarrassed as you might be, it's better than dealing with the damage that could happen if you don't seek medical attention. Avoid this worry altogether by using anal-safe toys.

Be realistic about the size. Bigger is not always better! Consider the size of objects that you've accommodated previously. Was it two fingers? A cock? A fist? A toy that is around the same size or slightly larger is reasonable, but making a jump from two fingers to a 2-inch-diameter butt plug is perhaps unrealistic. If you can afford it, get toys of many different sizes so you can work your way up from smaller to larger ones.

Many anal toys are made from nonporous silicone, glass, metal, plastic, or other similar materials. These are good choices because they're easy to clean and take care of. Some materials, like jelly rubber, PVC, vinyl, and some elastomers (also known as TPE and TPR) are porous, which means that bacteria can get trapped in the surface of the toy, even if you scrub it—in fact, some of the softer materials can be damaged by overly enthusiastic cleaning. Because these toys are so hard to clean, your best bet is to cover them with a condom every time.

It's probably a good idea to stick with objects that are meant to be used as sex toys, rather than using something you happen to have around the house. However, if you feel suddenly inspired, make sure that anything you use is smooth, has a base, and is either nonporous or (better) covered with a condom.

Realistic Expectations for Toys

We've spoken with some men who have had disappointing experiences with toys. In some cases, it may be that the toy wasn't right for them, but sometimes it's because they had unrealistic expectations about how the toy would feel. This is especially true for popular toys that work for a lot of men, such as the Aneros (which we describe later in this chapter).

Fans of the Aneros absolutely rave about it. They talk of having multiple orgasms over the period of an hour or more. Understandably, new Aneros users are probably hoping for similar fireworks. So they pop it in, follow the instructions on the package, wait eagerly for the magic, and wonder why nothing happens. They are expecting the toy to instantly create the pleasure all by itself. Like instant coffee—just add hot water and serve! But that's not how it works. Putting a sex toy into an unaroused anus is like pouring gasoline over firewood that hasn't been lit—you won't get anywhere if you don't have a match handy.

You have to light the fire first—get yourself aroused. Fantasize, watch porn, or read erotica, touching yourself in any way that you enjoy. Even if the ultimate goal is a hands-free prostate orgasm, you may get the best results from touching your cock for the first few times while you get used to the new toy. You might just need to slow down and relax enough to really feel what's happening rather than thinking about what you want to have happen. Once you are turned on, adding a toy is a great way to fuel the fire.

It's also good to remember that when it comes to sex, nothing works the same for everyone. You might follow all the instructions for a particular toy and discover that nothing happens. That doesn't mean that there's anything wrong with you, and it doesn't necessarily mean that the toy won't work for you if you try again another time. Some men discover that toys that didn't do much before drive them wild after they've gained some prostate experience.

Or you could chalk it up as an experiment that didn't go

the way you wanted and try something else. While it can be disappointing, don't take it personally. It just means that you need something else. Fortunately, there are lots of options.

BUTT PLUGS

Butt plugs come in a wide variety of shapes and sizes, but the basic design is: thin-thick-thin-thick, in that order. They start with a slender point of entry, followed by a thicker middle that sits inside the rectum, then a thin neck that the anal sphincters close around, and lastly a flared base that sits outside the anus for easy retrieval.

Most plugs don't give you much prostate stimulation—they are generally designed to go in and stay put, and aren't made for motion. Many of them do not go deep enough to sit along the prostate, and even if they do, they won't be doing much. But they are great for getting the ass warmed up for motion or larger toys. Also, they nicely bring attention to the prostate if you wear one for motion-oriented activities like being spanked or fucking someone.

Some plugs have a curved tip that looks like it would work for the prostate, and some of them do, especially if the flared base is shaped to hold it in the right position. But if your plug has a rounded base, it might rotate once you have it inserted, which will move the curve away from your prostate. If your plug has a curved tip and a vibrator in the base, it's more likely to work for prostate fun, since the vibration makes up for the lack of back-and-forth motion.

BEST OF BOTH WORLDS

Sometimes you want to be the one *doing* the fucking and have your prostate rubbed at the same time. Well, unless there is a third person present, this is likely too much of a contortion for most people to do with fingers. But the right toy could be just the ticket!

The important thing here is to choose a toy that stays in place without you having to hold it. Butt plugs are well suited for this, since they are designed to go in and stay put. Just make sure you choose a toy that is long enough to actually contact the prostate.

Unfortunately, some plugs have a tendency to fall out, especially during orgasm. This is much less likely if the bulb (the thicker part inside your body) is a good bit wider than the narrow neck. The closer the two are in size, the harder it'll be to keep it in. You may find that it is easier to keep the toy in place in some positions than in others, so do a little experimenting.

The Aneros is very popular for this purpose, since it has such a well-designed pivot action that presses the toy against your gland every time that you thrust your hips. Also, a vibrating plug can add a little zip.

MADE WITH THE PROSTATE IN MIND

There are lots of anal toys on the market, but most of them are not made with the specific intention of stimulating the prostate. Lately, however, there has been an upswing in the number of prostate-specific toys being manufactured. Toy companies seem to have noticed the trend and are expanding their product lines to meet the market demand. They are also increasingly addressing a market of straight men and male–female couples.

Aneros

The Aneros Company is one of the best-known prostate toy manufacturers. Its product, the Aneros, was originally designed as a medical device to facilitate prostate massage by making it easier to milk the prostate and "relieve congested prostate fluid."[17] Many patients reported unexpected and pleasant sexual side effects, and eventually the company began to market the product as a sex toy. The company has also developed other models in slightly different shapes and sizes to accommodate different body types and offer different sensations. The narrower version is easier for beginners to insert. The wider one spreads the sensation over more surface area, so it can actually feel less intense. And the company even has a model that includes a pulsing vibrator for that extra stimulation. Although nothing works for everyone, Aneros toys get rave reviews from a lot of men!

The Aneros is shaped like an upside-down *T*. It features a slender, gently curved insertion piece with a narrowed neck. When the Aneros is inserted, the front arm of the *T* rests outside the body, against the perineum, to press into the perineum point. The back arm serves as a handle, but you don't use the handle to move the toy inside you: the unique thing about the Aneros is that it is designed for hands-free motion.

To move the toy, you squeeze your PC muscles. (See chapter 6, Searching for the "Magic Button.") When you tighten these muscles, you pull the toy up and in. Since the front arm of the toy sits on the outside, nestled against the perineum, when your PC muscles pull the toy inward, this pressure on the front arm creates a lever effect, tipping the toy forward so it presses against the prostate. Each time you contract your PC muscle, whether you do it on purpose or out of reflex, the toy massages the prostate.

The pressure on the perineum can be too intense for some, especially when they first begin using it. If you're getting too much pressure, you can tape a cotton ball to the front arm to soften the intensity. Most users get accustomed to the pressure over time and then find it to be quite pleasurable.

To ensure that the end of the front arm sits over the right area on your perineum, find your "sweet spot" in advance, then measure the distance from your asshole and buy the right toy for your body according to the measurements listed online. It is also possible to (very gently!) bend the perineum arm slightly forward to elongate it. The perineum arm tends to slide off to one side rather than rest in the center, especially if your cock is hard. Just keep moving it back to center.

Since these toys are hands free, you can use your hands for other things like stroking your cock or washing the dishes. Plenty of people love to wear these toys while fucking someone else. Or you can move your hips from side to side to create a windshield wiper motion. There are lots of ways to experiment with these toys.

It can be tempting to use your hands to create the motion of the toy. You might find that pleasurable, but it's better to use the PC muscle; it helps jump-start your arousal. It's not just about moving the toy toward and away from the prostate: repeated tightening of the PC is what you do when you climax. Contracting and relaxing these muscles adds significantly to your arousal, wakes up the tissue, and is great exercise. A stronger PC makes for stronger orgasms, so this is a great way to get in shape. A significant part of the success of the Aneros is likely due to the added bonus of getting your PC in shape and the associated benefits. (See chapter 6, Searching for the "Magic Button.")

The manufacturer provides online forums where you can trade tips with other users, get advice, and discover new ways to enjoy your prostate. One thing—don't take another guy's instructions as law. Everyone is different, and you will need to experiment with a variety of positions to find what works best for you.

Nexus

The Nexus line of prostate toys has a design similar to the Aneros, basically an upside-down *T* with a handle to the back and a perineum arm to the front. In contrast, many of the Nexus toys have a rolling ball in the perineum arm that slides across the perineum rather than a tab that presses in.

The Nexus Vibro is very popular. The vibration is concentrated at the tip, instead of at the base as with many insertable vibrators, so more of the vibration goes to the prostate. (Not everyone likes vibration on their prostate, but some men love it.) The Vibro has different vibration speeds that seem to work very well for the prostate, according to many who have used the toy.

At the time of this writing, Aneros had recently sued Nexus for patent infringement, and they agreed to a settlement which dictates that Nexus will not be able to sell toys in the US for a certain period of time.

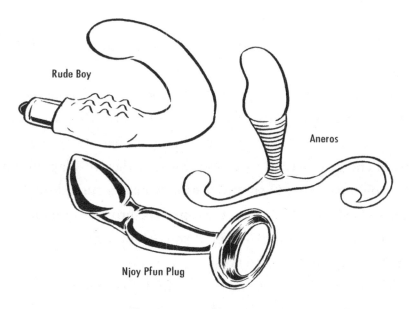

Rude Boy

Aneros

Njoy Pfun Plug

Illustration 22. Prostate Toys

Others

There are some other prostate-specific toys, like the Naughty Boy and the Rude Boy, made by Rock Chick. To use these, you sit on them and rock or gyrate your hips to create the motion.

Also check out Pure Plug, a line of shiny stainless-steel butt plugs that get good reviews for prostate stimulation. Make sure to pick one that is long enough to actually reach the gland. Start off in a in facedown position so that the weight of the toy is pressing into your prostate. Then try moving your hips to see what motion it creates.

G-SPOT TOYS

The road map to the prostate is pretty similar to that of the G-spot in women: enter the appropriate orifice, go in about 2–3 inches, point to the front of the body, and you're there. This means that plenty of toys made for one also work for the other. In fact, we've spoken with a number of men whose toy of choice is actually a G-spot toy that they've adapted for their own pleasure. G-spot toys usually have a curved tip that can be used to hook around the top of the prostate and milk it downward or press into it. And if you're looking for vibration, you'll surely find it in the G-spot toy section.

These toys often lack the tapered neck that many anal toys feature, which allows the anal muscles to hold a toy in place. But perusing G-spot toys will open a lot of options for you— because there are so darn many of them! Just make sure that your toy is anal safe: smooth, easy to clean (or else cover it with a condom), and with a flared base to keep it from slipping all the way in.

VIBRATORS

Vibrators are popular for anal play—they feel great and help relax the sphincter muscles. You might like vibrating prostate toys for the way they feel on the anus, for the prostate sensations, or both! It's worth noting that you might find the prostate vibration a little too intense or distracting, or it might make your orgasm amazing. The only way to find out is to try it.

When you're first looking for your prostate, we suggest not

using a vibrator (or at least not switching the vibration on), because vibration can make it a bit harder to isolate the prostate sensations and be sure you're in the right place. But once you're confident that you know where yours is, vibration can be a great addition.

Many battery vibrators are sold as novelty toys, which means they tend to break pretty quickly. While that's unfortunate, it does make them less expensive, so you can try a few different ones out without also breaking the bank. Once you know what you like, more durable (and generally more expensive) models are out there.

Besides durability, another factor that affects the price of your toy is what it's made of. Some materials are less expensive, but generally more difficult to clean. Others are more durable and are nonporous, but they tend to cost more. We'll discuss the common sex toy materials and how to take care of them later in this chapter.

Electric vibrators are much more durable than most battery models, but they're a bit bigger than you might want and, of course, you need to be near an outlet. If you want something for longer sessions, an electric toy like the Hitachi Magic Wand or the Wahl Coil vibrator might be a good bet.

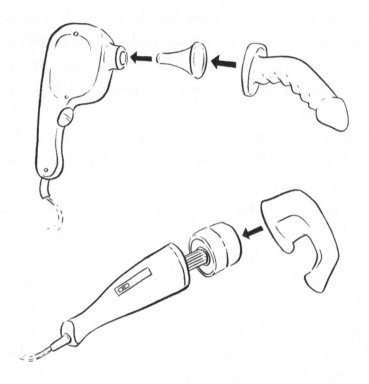

Illustration 23. Electric Vibes and Attachments: Wahl Coil with Suction Cup Attachment; Hitachi Magic Wand with G-Spotter Attachment

The intended purpose of electric vibrators is back massage, but there are some easy ways to make them work for sex.

Neither of the models in Illustration 23 should be inserted into the body, but you can use them to make an insertable toy vibrate. If you have a Hitachi Magic Wand, you can insert a dildo or plug into your anus and hold the head of the vibrator against it. Or you can purchase a G-spotter attachment, which slips over the head and has a curved shaft that's perfect for prostate fun. The Wahl Coil vibrator has an attachment that works like a suction cup. You can stick any silicone dildo with a flat base to it and have fun. With this combination the entire length vibrates, so you'll get anal and prostate pleasure. Silicone toys transmit vibration a lot better than softer materials like jelly rubber, so they work very well when used with an electric vibrator like this.

DILDOS

Dildos are long and more or less smooth, so they're well suited for an in-and-out motion. Some resemble a penis and others are less realistic. Choose a dildo with a curve for greater ease reaching the prostate, and make sure the inside of the curve is always facing the front of the body. The curve allows you to reach up and around the top of the prostate and press downward against it, like the "come hither" motion people like to use with finger massage. These models also work well for long in-and-out strokes, so the toy slides across the whole gland.

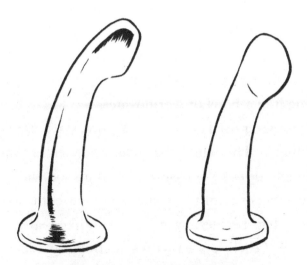

Illustration 24. Curved Dildos

For more direct pressure, try sitting on the toy and rocking back and forth; this works especially well with a midlength dildo, whose tip is at the prostate. Or reach your arm behind your ass and hold the base of the toy as you push it in toward the front of the body. Pushing in and out by curling your fingers and wrist can get tiring quickly, so try cupping the base of the toy in your hand and using the motion of your arm and shoulders to pivot it up and down so it presses against the prostate; or try an in-and-out motion.

If your dildo has a bulb at the end or a prominent head, it can be nice for hooking around the top of the prostate and milking it with a downward motion on the withdrawal stroke. If your toy has a very pronounced head or ridges, it can feel great but it might be too much on the sensitive anus. These models may not be good choices until you're familiar with anal play and know what you like.

In general, rigid materials such as glass, metal, or firm silicone make it easier to apply pressure. A dildo made of harder material will feel bigger than a softer dildo of the same size, so you may want to get a slimmer toy. Glass and metal tend to feel cold to the touch, but you can warm the toy up in advance by putting it in a bowl of warm water.

If you've never used an anal toy before, start off with something slimmer. The worst that could happen is that it's not wide enough to rock your world. But if it's too wide, it can be uncomfortable or painful, so don't let your enthusiasm make you go too big. Besides, even guys who like really large toys often start off each session with something smaller and work their way up, so having a slimmer toy is a good bet.

For prostate play, you probably don't need anything longer than six inches, but that's the short end of the range for most dildo makers. Don't worry, though. If it's longer than you like, you can simply hold it a bit further up the shaft and not insert the whole length.

STRAP-ON HARNESSES FOR HIM AND HER

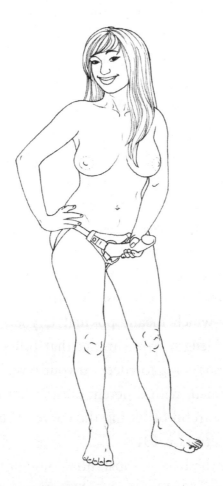

Illustration 25. Woman Wearing Strap-on Harness and Dildo

Using a dildo with a partner can be a lot of fun, whether handheld or with a harness. Going the handheld route gives a lot of control over smaller motions and changes in pressure and angle. But using a harness keeps everyone's hands free for other activities, and if you have a fantasy of getting fucked, there's nothing quite like a harness to make that work.

Pick Your Dildo First

The first thing to do is pick a dildo that works for you, then find a harness that will work with it. Look for one with a flat base for the harness ring to grasp. And since it'll probably be moving in and out, find one that's smooth instead of one with lots of bumps and ridges. While dildos with a pronounced head or curve work well as a handheld option, most people prefer a more gentle curve when using a strap-on harness.

For strap-on play, a slightly longer toy sometimes works better because you lose a little length to the harness and to the space between bodies. Also, many men who enjoy getting fucked really enjoy it when the object slides over the prostate, all the way in and all the way out. A shorter one can easily end up moving not *across* the prostate, but directly *into* the prostate—which means poking! If your dildo is about 4–6 inches in length, you can get that full-surface prostate stroking without going too deep. If your favorite dildo is a bit longer, experiment with different positions, and if you do go for depth, be careful of hitting the curve of the rectum. (See chapter 5, Penetration 101.)

Make sure the base is substantial enough for the harness to grasp. Some toys have bases that are too narrow for the ring to hold or so soft that they simply pull through and fall out. Some harnesses have the ring sewn in, so you can't change the size. In others, the ring is held in with snaps, so you can swap it out for a larger or smaller ring, which gives you a few more options.

Harness Selection

These days, there are lots of different harnesses out there. Some are leather, which looks and feels sexy, but they can't be 100 percent cleaned because leather is porous, so it's probably a good idea to use it with just one partner. Some are machine-washable fabric, which makes clean-up a snap. Check with the manufacturer or the store you purchase it from for cleaning instructions. For example, if it has nylon straps, don't put it in the dryer—it can melt! Some harnesses are frilly, some are no-nonsense, and some have sexy designs or colors. Take a look and find one that fits your personality and makes you feel sexy!

Many sex shops allow customers to try on harnesses over their clothes. If you live near a store, definitely take advantage of this opportunity: a snug fit is very important to having it work properly. A loose harness won't hold the dildo in place, so you won't be able to control the motion very well, and it might not look as sexy as it could. Wear snug pants so you can get a good feel for the harness. If you feel bashful, bring a close friend, and remember, people at the shop see this all day—it's nothing new to them. If you don't have a store near you, you can order a harness online. See the Resources for recommended retailers.

Harness Styles

There are three basic styles of strap-on harness: those that fit like a thong, those that fit like a jockstrap, and a few that fit like shorts or underwear.

Thong harnesses have one strap that goes between your legs. They give you the most control, but they feel like you're wearing a very tight pair of jeans; some people dislike the sensation. Plus, if the wearer wants to receive penetration as well as giving it, the strap is in the way.

The jockstrap style features two straps that go around the back of your upper thighs. They're more comfortable and give easy access to the wearer's genitals, if you want that. But they can take a little more practice to use, and if you change positions, you may need to adjust the straps.

Harnesses that are built like shorts or briefs look great, but be sure that they hold the dildo firmly. If the material stretches, your toy will hang downward and you'll have a lot less control over it.

Whatever model harness you choose, you want the base of the dildo to rest on your pubic bone. If it's up too high, on your abdomen, it will be harder to thrust. You can snug it down a bit lower so it rests over the clit, giving good clit stimulation and creating the feeling that the dildo is an extension of the clit.

Vibrating Dildos and Harnesses

Many sex shops carry dildos with a vibrator in the base to make the dildo vibrate. And some harnesses come equipped with a little pocket where you can insert a small bullet vibrator so that it sits over the clit. People who like vibrators often find that these give them a little extra stimulation, making the harness more fun. But these little vibes tend to be on the mild side, especially when the sensations have to travel through the material of the harness.

On his end, the vibration will be felt most strongly at the anal opening—which some men really enjoy—but it is not likely to be felt on the prostate. If you decide to try a vibrating dildo, make sure that the vibrator sits all the way inside the base of the dildo, so that the surface into which you will be pressing at the base of the dildo is flat and there isn't a little hard vibe poking out for you to bruise against.

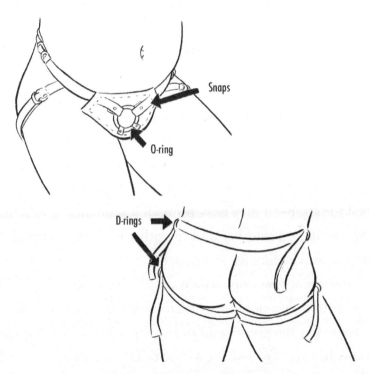

Illustration 26. Jockstrap-Style Strap-on Harness

Strap-on Double Dildos

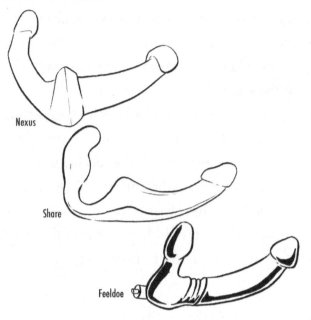

Nexus

Share

Feeldoe

Illustration 27. Strap-on Double Dildos

Traditional double dildos are long, straight toys that are basically two dildos connected at the base, forming one long, double-ended dildo. This is not the kind of double dildo used with a harness in strap-on play. The double dildos that are suited for strap-on play have more of a right angle, so that one end goes up and into her and the other end sticks straight out from the pelvis, like an erect cock.

There are a few popular toys with this design. The Nexus is one option, but don't confuse it with the Nexus line of prostate toys. On the giver's end of the toy, it's a dildo that curves up and inward toward the G-spot. The material is semifirm with a little give and comes in multiple sizes.

The Feeldoe and the Share are two other choices. These toys are different from the Nexus in that the giver's end, instead of a shaft, is shaped like a bulb. The bulb is meant to be held in by the vaginal muscles, though some women find it can be difficult to hold on to. The Feeldoe is quite firm, so it may feel like a lot for both partners—we recommend doing ample warm-up before using it and starting with gentle, controlled strokes. The Feeldoe, like the Nexus, comes in a variety of sizes.

The Share is fairly similar to the Feeldoe; it's a bit softer and it features a larger bulb, plus a clitoral ridge that comes up and over the clit and allows for some nice friction there. The bigger bulb makes it easier for the vaginal muscles to hold on to, but some people find it too wide for comfort.

Harness-Free Use

Because the Feeldoe and the Share have a bulb on the giver's end instead of a shaft, it is possible to use these toys without a harness, since the bulb provides something for the giver to clasp. This is great for those who are not fond of straps and prefer the more natural look of a woman who is fully nude except for the silicone cock sticking out from between her thighs.

However, using these toys without a strap-on takes some practice to master. The toy may fall out repeatedly when you first try this, especially if you are using it in a position where gravity is working against you. This is compounded by the fact that the receiving asshole might be very tight. These toys were generally designed with girl–girl pairs in mind and the ass tends to be tighter (and so gives more resistance) than a vagina.

If the woman has never been on the giving end of strap-on sex before, it's probably best to try it several times with the harness, and then see if you can go without. That way, she can learn to steer a cock and master the motion of fucking without also having to worry about keeping her end from falling out! You can always play without the harness later, if you prefer—though by holding the dick in place a harness makes many positions possible which would otherwise tend to cause the dick to fall out of her pussy.

When you would like to try it harness free, there are some positions that work better than others. Keeping your thighs together tends to help the toy stay in place. You can do this in missionary, cowboy, or doggy positions. Or, you can make gravity work for you by having the receiver lie on his belly with his legs together, and the giver straddling him, sitting or lying over him. In this position, you can probably open your legs without the toy falling out.

If you want to buy a harness to use with a Feeldoe or a Share dildo, make sure it is one that works with a double dildo. Most harnesses are designed to be used with regular dildos only; not all work with a double-ended toy. The usual construction involves a ring that you put the toy through and a backdrop cloth—a small piece of material that sits between the body and the base of the toy. In some harnesses there is a hole in this cloth so the harness can be used with a double dildo (assuming that the hole is big enough for the dildo to fit through it). In others, the cloth can be removed, leaving just the ring and straps—that works too. If the harness does not have a hole in the cloth and if the cloth cannot be removed, it can't be used with a double dildo.

INFLATABLES

A lot of guys like to start off their prostate play with a slim toy and work their way up to something bigger as they get more turned on. One great way to get this effect is by using an inflatable toy.

Inflatable toys are made of stretchy materials like latex. They come with a handheld pump so you can increase the size of the toy while it's inside you. These are often best for creating a pleasurable feeling of fullness in the ass, which many anal players enjoy, but they can also exert an agreeable pressure on the prostate by their sheer size. Since they apply pressure in every direction, they work best for someone who has experience with and enjoys larger sizes.

If you would like to tap into your prostate sensations while using an inflatable toy, get one that is deep enough to sit over the prostate—at least 4 inches. Start by inflating the toy so it is just firm enough to insert, and then adjust the size to whatever feels good. It can feel good to pump it up slowly, then deflate it, so that you can experience the inflation repeatedly. If you pump it very large, the tube might blow off the pump. This is annoying, but usually you can just put it back on and hold it in place with your thumb and forefinger while you use the toy.

Be sure to use plenty of lubricant. When you deflate these toys, the walls of the rectum slide over the latex as it shrinks.

If your lubricant has dried out, this can be pretty uncomfortable. A silicone lube might be the best way to go, since it won't dry out.

ELECTROSTIM

The Aneros isn't the only medical device that crossed over into the world of sex toys. Electricity stimulation (or "electrostim") toys are among them as well. Power boxes such as the TENS machine are commonly used for physical therapy to apply electric currents to the body via pads placed on the skin. These devices have been adapted to the world of sex by various toy manufacturers. For thrill-seeking prostate players, electrical toys can add a nice zing to your repertoire!

Electrostim is all about mixing arousal with the intense sensation of a mild electrical charge. Sound painful? It can be—in fact, some BDSM practitioners are drawn to it for just that reason. But it doesn't have to be. At a low setting it feels like a faint tingle. At higher levels it can feel like a throb or a zap. The sensations can often be felt through the skin in deeper levels of tissue, thus the electric charge of a well-placed metal butt toy can pass through the rectal wall to be felt in the prostate.

Electrostim is an advanced type of play; you should do lots of research before using these toys (not to mention investing in the expensive equipment!). In use, always make sure you put the control panel in a safe place, where no one will accidentally hit it and push the dial into high gear! Always turn the device off before removing or adjusting the connections to your body—if the electricity is still running when you reduce the surface area it is contacting, all the charge will be concentrated in that bit of skin, which can be more than you wanted.

URETHRAL SOUNDS

The urethral sound is yet another medical implement that has crossed over as a sex toy. Doctors use sounds to locate obstructions such as scar tissue in the urethra. These smooth, slender rods of stainless steel are inserted into the urethra to stretch it gently, reducing obstructions and allowing free flow of urine. Some people use urethral sounds as sex toys.

If this rather painful-sounding description is making you wonder why anyone would do this, it's good to remember that when it's done carefully it can be a lot of fun. The insertion of the cool steel rod and the gentle stretching of the urethra can feel good. And, what is most relevant to us here: once you're in deeper than the base of the penis, it's possible to gently guide the tip of the sound through the portion of the urethra running through the center of the prostate.

Some who have experienced this describe a wave of pleasure that comes over them when the tip is in contact with the prostate. At that depth, subtle (we mean really subtle!) movements of the sound can be felt in the prostate, with great pleasure. Some recommend rotating the sound—how much you can do this depends on the shape of the sound—or gently tapping the base to transmit vibrations, or slowly moving it in and out a bit. Any movement of the sound, whether during insertion, removal, or when stimulating any of your internal parts, should be done very slowly and gently—it is easy to cause serious damage.

For erotic play, most guys use a set of sounds, starting with smaller ones and working up to larger sizes. The increasing size creates a stretching sensation in the urethra which many enjoy. Sounds come in a few different shapes—some gently curved, some straight. The urethra takes a gentle curve upward at the level of the prostate, but not as dramatically as portrayed in many anatomy diagrams. When a sound is fully inserted, the angle is about 55 degrees from the laid-out body (if a hard cock sticking straight up in the air is at 90 degrees). Interestingly, taking it out can feel a bit more daunting than inserting. To insert, you just allow the weight of the toy to do the work, whereas with the withdrawal, you are actively pulling outward, and you have to be careful of the angle so that you aren't putting too much pressure downward toward the perineum. It is important never to force the sound and to gently follow the direction of the urethra.

Be warned that when you insert a sound, you are giving any bacteria on that metal rod a free ride deep into the urethra. It could result in a urinary tract infection, a bladder infection, or prostatitis, so use a careful and stringent sterilization method. Also, the metal is hard and heavy, so you must be very careful not to puncture your partner internally by pushing too hard. If you have a faint tinge of pink in your urine after using a sound, that's not likely to be an issue. However, if at any point you have large amounts of blood flowing out of the tip of the cock, get to an emergency room.

Urethral sounds are a very advanced type of prostate play

and require a lot of skill to be used safely. The best way to learn how to use them is with someone who has personal experience. At the very least, do your research—there's quite a bit of good information online. We've described the basics, but you'll need more to do it safely, so get the info you need first.

TOY MATERIALS AND CLEANING

Other than sounds, most toys you might use for prostate play are designed for anal use. There are a few basic tips you should know about taking care of them.

These days, many sex toys are made from high-quality, nonporous materials: stainless steel, borosilicate glass, silicone, hard plastic, intramed, and even sealed wood. Any of these toys can be washed with soap and water, and many of them can be disinfected in boiling water for five minutes, in the top rack of a dishwasher, or even in a 10 percent bleach solution for 15 minutes. (Wash the bleach off afterward.) Check the information that comes with your toy.

Certain materials are somewhat porous. Jelly rubber, soft plastic, vinyl, PVC, elastomer, and silicone blends generally can't be boiled without melting and they often develop small pockets in the surface which can trap bacteria. Since cleanliness is more of an issue for anal play than some other types of sex, it's a good idea to cover these toys with a condom—then you can just take off the condom and rinse off the lubricant. Be sure to roll the condom all the way over the base to ensure that the entire toy is covered.

Some people use antibacterial soaps for their toys. While

these products can be useful, most people don't use them correctly. The most common antibacterial ingredient is triclosan, which must be left on the surface for two minutes to have the desired effect. If you don't soap up and let the toy sit for two minutes before rinsing it off, you might as well use any regular soap. When exposed to UV light, triclosan converts to dioxin, a dangerous chemical, and in any case, research has shown that regular soap is just as effective as the antibacterial kind. Simply wash with soap and hot water for 15 seconds and you'll be all set.

12

ANAL SEX AND STRAP-ON FUCKING

For many men, the preferred method of giving the prostate a little rubdown is to be on the receiving end of anal sex with a cock or a strap-on dildo. A number of anal sex positions angle the cock or dildo so that it slides over the prostate with each in-and-out motion, giving a hands-free massage. Even in other positions in which the prostate is not in perfect alignment with the cock, it still gets some pressure (since there is pressure in all directions when you are being filled up) and some jostling (since the whole pelvis may be jostled by the thrusting motion).

If your ass is ready for this level of stimulation, and you have a trusted partner with an appropriately sized cock or dildo, anal sex offers an entirely different experience from prostate massage with fingers. In fact, some even prefer it over finger play. By virtue of being thicker than fingers, cocks and (many) dildos apply more pressure in all directions, including pressure on the prostate—which can add to your pleasure. Because the force is not all concentrated behind a small fingerpad, the stimulation is broader over the surface of the prostate. This lesser concentration might leave some wanting, but for others for whom the very direct, focused pressure of a finger massage is too much, the broad in-and-out strokes of a cock or dildo sliding over it may be just the ticket. And the bouncy, jostling motions of fucking can really feel amazing on the gland.

The prostate is not the *only* thing that makes receptive anal sex pleasurable for a man. But for many men who love anal sex, the prostate is a significant part of the pleasure they experience, even though some may not realize that what they are feeling is their prostate.

Some men first discover their prostate gland accidentally, before they have even heard about it, while exploring anal sex. One fellow describes his experience of this: "My playmate liked to use her strap-on and I quickly discovered that some positions felt *much* better than other ones. I didn't realize that this was my prostate at first. In fact, I don't exactly recall when I made the connection[...]."

Though many men feel amazing prostate stimulation while getting fucked, it's not going to happen for every man, every time. The same is true for women: not all women feel their G-spot activated every time they have vaginal sex. Remember from chapter 7, Find It: Locating the Gland, that it is possible to press directly over your partner's prostate and not have him feel anything remarkable. Some men simply may not feel a great deal of prostate sensation during anal sex. Of course, we believe that it is possible to learn to tune in to the prostate through practice.

DISCLAIMER: For the sake of simplicity, we use the terms *dildo* and *cock* interchangeably in this chapter. Some of you will be playing with a flesh cock, others with a manufactured cock—but really, if we spent the whole chapter saying "cock or dildo" it would get a little tedious, wouldn't it?

A Different Way of Doing the Same Thing

Some male–female couples are happy to explore anal play with fingers and toys but feel that anal intercourse is a different matter. For some, this is because strap-on fucking is seen as too closely resembling anal intercourse between gay men, or sex with the man playing the "woman's role."

If you are having these concerns, first we'd invite you to consider: Is there any real difference between using a toy by holding it in your hand versus attaching it to your pelvis or thigh? Either way, you are creating the motion of the toy. We invite you to look at it as a different way of doing the same thing: pleasuring the prostate. If issues about masculinity are coming up, we recommend that you check out chapter 13, Real Men Don't, for an in-depth discussion of these concerns.

TECHNIQUE

Anal intercourse inherently involves a lot of in-and-out motion. This is different from finger massage, which consists of smaller movements. Because of the emphasis on motion, it is imperative that you use lots of lube. If you don't use enough, there will be too much friction and it will likely become uncomfortable very quickly.

Anal sex is often perceived as a pinnacle sex act. Often when someone gets the idea to have anal intercourse the impulse is to say, "Okay, great! Put it in my ass right now!" A severe ass pounding is the stuff of many a fantasy, but no matter how hot that fantasy is for you, it is important that you don't rush into it before you are ready.

It is highly unrealistic to expect to have pleasurable anal sex during your first attempt at anal penetration. We've heard lots of stories about painful, entirely pleasureless anal sex experiences. This is where many of them come from: eager newbies who rush to anal intercourse before they've learned how to warm up. Ideally, you should only attempt anal fucking after you've practiced penetration with reasonably sized objects—and liked it—several times. This is one of the best ways to ensure that you get the pleasurable experience you are hoping for.

The ass doesn't do well with a zero-to-60 approach, especially for beginners. So for best results, take the time to get the ass ready. By way of a warm-up, give yourself a gentle prostate massage with your fingers. This awakens the prostate early in the session, so that by the time you get to anal sex it will be perked up and eager to revel in the persistent strokes of the cock over it. The more stimulation the prostate gets *before* intercourse, the more it will be able to generate sensation *during* intercourse, since it will be that much more swollen and aroused. Once you are warmed up, open your ass slowly, moving from smaller to larger objects and allowing plenty of time for it to adjust between insertions. Use fingers or small toys before you take on that fat purple dildo!

Sometimes people rush anal sex because that's what they've seen in porn movies. While those movies can be lots of fun, they don't show sex the way it really works. Using porn for sex ed is like learning gun safety from watching an action film. In porn movies you almost never see any warm-up before anal sex, or anyone applying lubricant. Both of these steps happen before the cameras are turned on, to convey a fantasy about the immediacy of anal sex. So feel free to use these movies as inspiration, as long as you remember to do it differently in the bedroom.

Riding the Curve

If you are working with a curved cock, you are at an advantage. The curve allows the cock to reach up and around the top of the prostate on each instroke, so that it tugs downward on the prostate during the outstroke. This mimics the "come-hither" motion that is so popular in finger massage. Make sure that the inside of the curve is always facing the prostate. If the cock curves downward, favor rear-entry positions, and if it curves upward, favor face-to face positions.

Of course, if you are using a strap-on dildo, you can simply rotate the dildo in the harness so that it points up or down, according to your needs. Sometimes, with all the motion of fucking, the dildo migrates a little off to one side or the other, rotating in the harness so that the curve no longer leans toward the prostate. This is less likely to happen if you have a harness that holds the dildo snugly in place (with the appropriate size O-ring—see chapter 11, Toys). But even with a well-fitted ring, it can sometimes shift if it's a very vigorous fuck.

The trouble is, when you are inserted and the top half of the dick is buried in his ass, it is often difficult to tell which way the curve is facing without pulling out. The bases of dildos are usually round, so looking at the base won't help. For this reason, a dildo with a nonrounded base is your friend—you always know which way the curve is facing just by looking at the base of the dildo.

If you are using a toy with a circular base, there is a simple solution: put on the harness with the dildo, angle the toy the way you want it, and draw a line or a small mark on the base of the toy with a permanent marker to indicate which end is up. Flip the toy around and mark the other side too, for positions in which you want it curving in the opposite direction. (Do this in advance so the ink has time to dry completely.) To check whether it is still facing the right direction during penetration, all you have to do is glance down at your mark and adjust if necessary.

Finding the Angle

Often when you ask someone how to touch the prostate during anal sex, they simply say, "Just point toward the front of the body." This is true: when you are aiming for the prostate, you are always aiming toward the front of the body. However, there are a few pitfalls that you can watch out for.

If you didn't know better, you might "point toward the front of the body" in such a way that you direct your cock straight into the prostate, so that all the force of each stroke impacts the prostate head-on. As we mentioned in chapter 9, Prostate Massage, most men find poking sensations to be unpleasant, and this is likely to feel like a lot of poking.

Depending on the preferences of your partner, you may be able to do some nice things with this angle: it might feel good to have the head of a cock apply very gentle head-on pressure if it's only small, quick, jostling stokes (almost like a vibration) or very subtle pressure-on, pressure-off strokes. But any hard or forceful pressure you apply directly to the prostate is likely to feel like a poke: uncomfortable and overstimulating.

So don't jab it with the head of your cock like a battering ram breaking through a fortress door. Instead, use your cock to slide across it. This means changing the angle so that the force of the stroke is not directed *into* the prostate, but *along* it. You want the cock to apply a grazing pressure as it slides in and out over the prostate. This tends to work best with long strokes: all the way past it on the instroke so the head of the cock is beyond the prostate, and all the way past it again on the outstroke so that the head of the cock drags down along the whole surface of the gland.

Though these are long strokes, they don't need to be deep strokes. You need only go just past the prostate so that you can come down over it again on the outstroke (about 5 inches deep). If you have a longer cock, you may find that it is not necessary to insert it all the way. In fact, you may be better off not inserting it to its full length on each stroke. Which brings us to our second pitfall: hitting the first curve of the rectum.

As we described in chapter 5, Penetration 101, the rectum is not a straight line. Rather, it has a gentle *S* curve. In the book *Anal Pleasure and Health,* Jack Morin points out that if you angle the penetrative object too strongly toward the front of the body and then plunge deep, the tip of the object is likely to slam into the first curve during the instroke. This will be painful, especially if there is force behind it.

This is especially relevant when you are shooting for the prostate, which necessitates a forward angle to your fucking. To avoid hurting your partner by poking into the first curve of the rectum, be sure that when changing from shallower to deeper strokes you go softly at first; if you do hit the first curve, there won't be force behind your thrust. Take a moment to adjust the angle, gently feeling your way. Check in with him, or watch for signals of discomfort. The new angle will be less dramatically pointed toward the front of the body, so it may not deliver as much sensation to the prostate. However, switching from shallow to deep strokes and back again can be a nice change, and is a good way to give the prostate a break so that it doesn't get overstimulated.

Pivot

For variety, stop the in-and-out motion and do a little up-and-down pivot with your hips. For this, you use your cock like a seesaw. Insert about 4 inches of the shaft so that the cock is contacting the whole surface of the prostate, and gently move your hips in a subtle up-and-down motion. As your hips go up, the head of your cock will point down, putting pressure on the prostate. This mimics the "come-hither" curl that you would do with your fingers to milk the prostate.

This one works well in rear entry or missionary (with his ass is propped up on a pillow and you on your knees), or if he's in a sling and you are standing. For rear entry, you are pressing the head of the cock downward against the prostate by pivoting your hips upward. Likewise, in missionary positions, you are pressing the cock up into the prostate by pivoting your hips downward. Note that this is not a big motion. You don't lift your hips up or down more than an inch or so at a time.

In many positions, the receiver can create this effect himself: you insert to the right depth and he rocks his hips, curling toward the pubic bone and then unfurling the tailbone to nestle the head of the cock against the area he favors. This way, he can very specifically line you up to where he wants you.

Circle Hips

In a glorious union of the in-and-out stroke and the up-down pivot, you can move your hips in a circular motion as you fuck him. Basically, you just fuck him in and out while moving your hips upward on one stroke and downward on the other. Note: we are not talking about a circle that involves moving your hips right to left. That might feel good for the prostate too if you get the right angle, but the circle we're describing is the up-down motion. The idea is that you are dragging the head of the cock dramatically across the surface of the prostate with every outstroke.

Let's say he's lying on his back, his ass propped up with a pillow and his knees pulled in to his chest. You are kneeling, penetrating his ass. Now imagine a clock on your right hip: point to 12:00 and trace your finger clockwise around the clock. This is the motion that your hips will follow—instroke, pivot down, outstroke, pivot up. Now, remember the seesaw? As you are pulling out and simultaneously moving downward (3:00 to 6:00), the head of your cock seesaws up and strokes across the surface of the prostate.

This can be a tricky motion and may take some practice— definitely slow it down and build from lesser to greater speeds. Also, it really doesn't have to be a big motion: just enough to reach beyond the prostate, stroke along it on the outstroke, and push in again. If you were entering him from behind, you would simply move your hips in a counterclockwise motion (if the clock is on your right hip)—but you are always dragging across the prostate on the outstroke so you contact it from top to bottom (going with the natural flow of the glands it contains) and to avoid poking it.

Switch It Up

As always, variety is good. Vary the speed, rhythm, length of stroke, and depth of stroke. After a few prostate-focused strokes, change the angle and go deeper for a few strokes that don't focus so strongly on the prostate. Occasionally backing off from the gland not only prevents it from getting bored or overstimulated, but also allows the prostate to enjoy the contrast between right-on-it strokes and just-gliding-past-it strokes. It gives the gland a chance to recharge and to crave the attention, so when you return to it, it will be eager for more.

REMEMBER THE SWEET SPOT

In many positions, you can reach with your hand to apply pressure to his perineum and massage his sweet spot while you fuck him. This applies pressure to the prostate from two directions simultaneously, and the dual approach can feel really amazing. There is a sense of unification of the pleasure, activating a wider range of nerves.

In missionary positions, simply reach down with your thumb. In rear entry, you might externally rotate your hand (so the thumb points away from your body), then press into his perineum with the pads of your curled fingers. Just be careful not to dig your nails into his skin!

POSITIONS

Positions make a big difference in how much prostate stimulation you get. Experiment with different positions and different angles and discover with your partner what works best for the unique pairing of your bodies.

Rear Entry

Rear-entry positions are especially good for pleasuring the prostate. Lots of people have mentioned that they feel it the most in these positions. When you enter him from behind, it is very easy to direct the cock toward the front of the body. The head of the cock is ideally situated to slide across the prostate on the in-and-out strokes. And as a bonus, you can give him a reach-around! Rear-entry positions don't favor eye contact, but if you want to see your partner's face, you can position yourselves in front of a mirror.

On all fours (doggy style)

- He is on his hands and knees and you are behind him.

- Great freedom of motion for him. He can move his hips back and forth to meet the thrusts, rock his hips up and down, and adjust easily to get the right angle.

- Easy to line up the height. He can spread his legs wider or bring them together to adjust the height of his ass so it lines up with your cock.

Doggy style with head down

- He is on his elbows and knees, with his face lowered to the bed so that the torso-to-thigh angle shifts from 90 degrees to 45 degrees.

- Changing the angle of the torso to the legs produces a subtle internal shift that positions the prostate closer to the surface: the prostate moves dorsally (toward the spine) and posteriorly (toward the anal opening).

- Have him lie over a pile of pillows so he won't have to work so hard to support himself with his arms. Some companies like Liberator make cushions that are specifically designed for sex. They're firm enough to give plenty of support, and the washable cover makes clean-up easy.

On his belly

- He lies flat on his belly, with you lying on top of him (between his legs) or kneeling upright (straddling his legs).

- Prop his ass up with a pillow for better accessibility.

Spoons

- Both partners lying on their sides, his back to your front, like two spoons nestled together in the silverware drawer.

- For better access, he can draw his top knee up so his thigh is perpendicular to his torso.

Bent over

- He is standing up and bending over, with his hands or elbows bracing him against the wall or a piece of furniture.

Missionary

Missionary positions have the receiver lying on his back and the giver approaching him from the front. These positions tend to be very comfortable for the receiver, letting him relax and lie back. Also, since he doesn't need his hands to hold himself up, he can use them to jerk off.

On his back

- When he is flat on his back, his asshole is not easily accessible. It becomes more accessible with a pillow under his hips: this makes it easier to get to his anus, and also allows for better angles.

- You can lie or kneel between his legs.

- He can bend his legs with his feet flat on the bed, or he can draw them up toward his chest. You can also put them over your shoulder, though this can be tiring.

- Position his legs at right angles to the body to soften the curves of the rectum, making it straighter and easier to penetrate without hitting the curves.[18] Bring his legs up closer to his chest to compress the pelvic area, adding to the pressure on the prostate.[19]

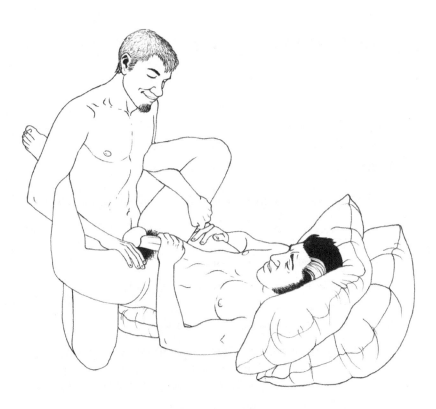

Illustration 28. Holding His Legs Up

WHAT TO DO WITH HIS LEGS

In missionary positions, you have greater access if his legs are drawn up, but that generally means either the receiver needs to hold them up with his hip flexors (which can be tiring) or one of you has to hold them up with your hands. Here are a few ways of doing it:

- He uses his arms to hold his own legs up, with his hands or (if he is flexible) his elbows wrapping behind the knees, or his hands holding his feet.

- You drape his legs over your shoulders.

- He pulls his knees to his chest, then you lie over them, putting some of your weight on the back of his thighs, with your hands on the bed at either side.

- He wraps his legs around your torso and puts his feet behind your mid-back. You slip your hands *under* his calves (supporting them) and *over* his thighs. Use your hands to pull his thighs toward you, your forearms to support his calves, and your elbows to keep his feet tucked behind you. (See Illustration 28.)

- You can improvise a seated sling position with a yoga strap. Connect the ends so that it forms a loop. He puts the loop around both of his legs, just above the knees. He lies back and pulls his knees to his chest. Then he grabs both pieces of the looped strap from between his knees and puts them behind his neck, so that his legs are supported. This can put a lot of strain on his neck; it helps if he has a pillow under his head and he positions the strap low on the neck. To help distribute the force evenly over the back of the neck, place a folded towel or small pillow between his neck and the straps. (See Illustrations 29–30.)

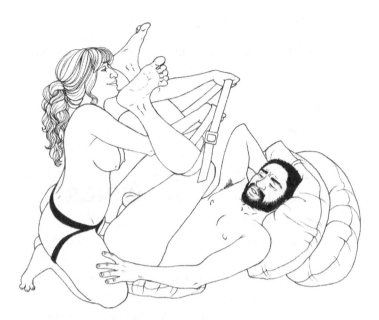

Illustration 29. Improvised Portable Sling, Step 1

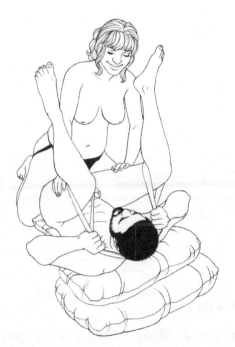

Illustration 30. Improvised Portable Sling, Step 2

Off the side of the bed or other furniture

- Position him on the edge of a bed or a desk, and stand or kneel (as your height dictates) on the floor.

- Don't do this on any furniture that may not safely hold his weight!

SLINGS AND SWINGS

Slings are immensely popular for anal sex, because they allow positioning that is both greatly comfortable and easy-access. A sling is, essentially, a little sex hammock that you hang from the ceiling. They are often made of leather but can be found in some other sturdy materials as well. The receiver lies on his back in the sling, with his ass hanging slightly off the edge and his knees pulled up toward his chest. You can also buy leg loops to attach to either side so the receiver can relax his legs.

This laid-back and fully supported position is ideal for anal sex because it really lets you relax fully, so your pelvic musculature can release and the ass can open more easily. The height of the sling can be adjusted before you get in it so that your ass is perfectly positioned to line up with your partner's pelvis when they are standing. They only need to point the cock inward and upward, and the prostate is right there waiting! Slings are spendy, generally ranging from $250 to $500, depending on the material, but it's a good investment. If you get a nice one and take good care of it, it'll last for years.

Cowboy (Receiver on Top)

- You lie down on your back and he climbs on top of you, straddling your cock.

- He can face toward or away from you. (This choice may depend on the shape of the cock—whether it curves upward or downward.)

- He can control the motion by bouncing up and down or gyrating on the cock.

- He can easily get it where he wants it by adjusting the depth and angle.

- Cowboy positions help him feel in control and help you feel assured that you are not going to hurt your partner.

- You can stroke him if he is facing toward you.

PEGGING: STRAP-ON SEX FOR GUY–GIRL COUPLES

Pegging is a recently coined term for an increasingly popular sexual practice: strap-on sex for male–female couples, with the man on the receiving end of penetration. Certainly, not every hetero couple is doing this, but an increasing number are trying it out, as shown by the emergence (and marketability!) of a number of products for this kind of play.

In 1998, a sex ed video on this subject titled *Bend Over Boyfriend* came out, and over the years it has sold well, generating a sequel. "Bend over boyfriend" or BOB for short has become a common term for this kind of sex. More recently, in 2009, Tristan Taormino released an educational video titled *Expert Guide to Anal Pleasure for Men*. In 2012 she came out with her follow-up, *Expert Guide to Pegging: Strap-on Anal Sex for Couples.*

Anecdotally, sex shop workers have reported an increase in guy–girl pairs shopping for butt toys for him, including strap-on harnesses and dildos. There are even "beginner strap-on kits" at sex shops that market to these pairs.

Some couples have a strong sense of reservation at the idea of pegging: they may have enjoyed experimenting with fingers and handheld toys, but strap-on sex feels like another ball game entirely. There is a feeling that anal intercourse is just *different* from other forms of anal play—too close in its association with the stigmatized realms of homosexuality or dominance and submission.

These concerns are common and it's often best to just talk it over openly with your partner. The way we see it, if she is making him feel good with her fingers, or with a toy held in her fingers, it's no different to do so with a toy attached to her pelvis. Inherently, the act is the same: she is pleasuring him (and hopefully enjoying herself too).

If you can get past the hang-ups, strap-on sex can be a way-hot experience for both the lady and the fellow she's givin' it to. First, it requires a great deal of trust for him to let her in this way, so it can foster deep feelings of intimacy; he is entrusting her with a part of himself that not a lot of men share with others, allowing himself to be vulnerable.

Then there's the excitement of trying something new together, of exploration and discovery. Plus the psychological turn-on of doing something naughty and taboo: the neighbors would flip if they knew, and that just makes it even hotter!

(Actually, the neighbors are probably doing it too.)

Also, the role reversal can be an eye-opening and memorable experience. Each partner gets to experience the other side of what they are used to: he gets to experience being on the receiving end of penetration, and she gets to be on the giving end. For that matter, quite a few women who have tried strap-on harnesses for the first time say that they now get how much work and responsibility fucking someone can be—and they don't even have to worry about their erections getting soft or reaching orgasm too soon!

And, of course, there is the actual physical pleasure it gives him, from the anal attention and the prostate. Many men find that receiving strap-on sex is an entirely different experience from other forms of anal play, and they appreciate the unique sensations it offers their prostate.

But this doesn't have to be all about him! Many women can get clitoral stimulation during strap-on sex if they position the base of the dildo over the clit. Some can even climax this way. There are also double dildos available that penetrate both partners simultaneously, so she can get vaginal stimulation while she fucks him.

Some eroticize the idea of power exchange that is suggested by penetration and play it up with fantasy and dominance/submission role play. For others, there is no suggestion of power exchange, and the approach can be playful and sensual instead: no D/s dynamic here; just some sweet lovin' for his whole body—no parts excluded.

Certainly, any kind of penetration can be delivered with a tone of dominance, but it is not inherently so. You may find that you and your partner like it both ways, and you can vary your approach nightly as the mood strikes you.

Finding Your Rhythm

Many women are not used to the fucking motion of the hips, so wielding a strap-on can be a bit awkward at first. Definitely don't build up a huge "I'm going to take your ass like a bandit" fantasy in advance of your first attempt at wielding a strap-on. You may find that you are not able to be as smooth in practice as you were in his and your shared fantasy.

When you're new, expect a learning curve. Many women, when they take on the role of the penetrator, are using muscles that they may not normally use in this way, so it may take some practice before you can fuck as smoothly as your boyfriend, who has probably had years of experience. Don't try to give him a fast and riotous pounding right away. If you are trying to move faster than your unpracticed muscles can coordinate, your strokes will be erratic and the angle will be changing with each stroke—which will feel about as good to his prostate as a flopping fish. Instead, take it slow and learn how to get a steady rhythm going. Once you've got that down, you can increase your speed. For each new position, start slow again and allow your muscle memory to develop through practice.

When you first enter him, hold the base of the dick in your hand to guide it in. You can hold still and have him back up onto it, or you can instruct him to "bear down" to open his sphincters. (See chapter 5, Penetration 101.) Don't shove all the way in right away—after the head pops in, hold still for a spell and let his ass get used to it before you work your way in deeper.

How She Can Get Off on Strap-on Play

Some women really love strap-on fucking their men—and not just because it's hot to watch him enjoy himself or because it's a hot fantasy to bend him over. As mentioned above, some women can experience real physical gratification from the act. All that thrusting and banging against his ass can give her some very nice friction on her clit—enough friction for some women to climax.

To maximize this sensation, wear the harness low, and position the dildo so that the base sits over the clit and the shaft extends out as if it were, itself, an extension of the clit. If you find the friction to be too much, try wearing panties under the harness. This softens the friction while also decreasing the likelihood that your genitals will come in contact with the ample quantity of lube which you are, of course, generously applying to the dildo.

Different positions work better for different women, but definitely try a position that lets you get in touch with the thrusting motion. If you have never come this way before, try really slowing down your strokes and tuning in to the way your clit feels. You might even practice by grinding on a pillow, or on his thigh. Dildos that maximize this effect are those with more to rub against—try one with a pair of balls attached, providing a larger surface area to grind on. Get one that is firm enough to allow easy fucking, but not so firm that it hurts to press into it.

And of course, there are plenty of dildos on the market that work for strap-on style sex but that penetrate the giver as well as the receiver. For info on these, as well as general tips for purchasing a strap-on harness, read up on toys in chapter 11.

REAL MEN DON'T

DOES IT MAKE ME LESS OF A MAN?

Many people have the idea that receiving penetration is in conflict with masculinity. The basic story goes like this: *Real men don't get fucked*—that's for women, fags, and sissies. Because receiving penetration is usually viewed as the woman's role in sex, a man may be worried that he isn't fulfilling the man's role if he takes a turn catching instead of pitching.

Thanks to the common (though incorrect) belief that the only men who like to receive anal penetration are gay men, many people think that if a man likes to be penetrated, he must secretly be gay. And it is also a common belief that being gay = being feminine = not very masculine.

Further, some people view penetration as an act of

domination, so a man may worry that he is being dominated if he lets his partner penetrate him—again, not a very "manly" thing to do.

All this contributes to the idea that if a guy opens his ass to some love, it makes him less of a man. To be clear, we think this is nonsense. But many men have a very real fear that if they receive penetration, they forfeit their masculinity. Needless to say, this can be a major roadblock to exploring and enjoying the prostate!

While not all men or their partners experience these concerns as a barrier to enjoying prostate play, it happens often enough that it's worth taking a closer look at these issues. In this chapter, we explain where these ideas come from, how they limit men, and why they aren't true.

THE "ACT LIKE A MAN" BOX

What does it mean to be a *"real* man," anyway? Although there's a lot of variation in how people define masculinity, some trends are pretty common. One of the best ways to describe these patterns is the "Act Like a Man" Box, which we first heard about in Paul Kivel's book *Men's Work: How to Stop the Violence That Tears Our Lives Apart.*

When people are asked to name the characteristics of a "real man" they usually come up with a pretty consistent list:

tall

strong

muscular

25–45 years old

able-bodied

heterosexual

cisgender[20]

competitive

dominant

cop

firefighter

mechanic

lawyer

businessman

CEO

caretaker

competent

leader

drinks alcohol

watches and plays sports

plays poker with his buddies

doesn't show emotions other than anger, excitement

stoic

violent

always wants sex

has lots of sexual partners

sex is about scoring

has a big penis

gets hard when he wants to

stays hard

gives his partner an orgasm (or multiple orgasms)

ejaculates when he wants to

sex is focused on intercourse, blow jobs (receiving), possibly anal (giving)

Now, the point needs to be made that not everyone shares these values or thinks highly of this kind of masculinity. Different cultures, communities, and families have different expectations around how they think men are supposed to act, and not everyone is in favor of this particular version of what it means to be a "real man." In fact, quite a lot of people would disagree with the valuation that emerges from the list above. Based on these characteristics, he's not necessarily a very nice guy!

But what's important about this list is that it shows how prevalent this particular "real man" ideology is. These ideas and images are so pervasive that even people who don't agree with them are still familiar with them. In fact, lots of people who don't agree that men should be violent and stoic still picture such a man when they hear the expression "a real man." So even if a guy didn't hear these messages from his family while growing up, odds are that he's absorbed them to some degree, simply because of how prevalent they are in the larger culture.

In communities where the "real man" ideal is in effect, it is a standard that men are measured and judged against. The degree to which a man conforms to these expectations is understood as an indicator of his value as a person. Other men may praise him for having these characteristics, or pass judgment on him for lacking them. And plenty of women learn these ideas, so sometimes they reinforce them too. Men absorb these ideas and judge themselves accordingly, even if they may not agree with these values rationally. This is called internalized judgment.

OUTSIDE THE BOX IS A SCARY PLACE

When people are asked to come up with some of the names that men get called when they don't meet the expectations of being a "real man," the responses are also pretty consistent:

gay	sissy	loser	wimp
fag	weak	bitch	maricón[22]
girl	punk[21]	pussy	poof

It's easy to see that it's a scary place outside the Box! Men who are perceived in these ways are subject to serious harassment, ostracism, and physical violence. Even if you've never been on the receiving end of this kind of treatment, we would bet that almost every man has seen it or heard about it happening to another person, especially when they were young. It's not surprising that so many men are concerned about keeping their masculinity points up.

Fortunately, more men than ever are realizing that although staying in the Box may keep them safe in some ways, it also limits them and keeps them from exploring and expressing their genuine selves.

IT ISN'T JUST GUYS

Some men with female partners might discover that while none of these beliefs are getting in their own way, their partner is having difficulty letting go of them. After all, it isn't just guys who can get caught up in the "Act Like a Man" Box. Quite a few women discover that they've absorbed judgments about how men, especially their partners, should behave. They might think that they've let go of the Box mentality but find that it's coming up during or after prostate play. The Box can be really hard to shake, especially since many of us start learning its traits when we're really young. Plus, sometimes when we try something new or challenging, our worries or anxiety bring old fears back to the surface even if we think we've shed them.

WHY THE BOX IS NONSENSE
You Can't Win

One of the characteristics of the Box is that it's very much an either/or. Even if you have many of the characteristics that are inside the Box, lacking any one of them can be taken to mean that you aren't a "real man." But it's almost impossible to have all the traits all the time. In fact, for all men, there will be a part of their lives when they are excluded from the Box because the "real man" image paints a picture of a man around age 25–45 years old, so any man outside that age range can't make the cut. Likewise, men with disabilities can never be in the Box. And some guys are simply not going to be tall or muscular.

To make it even harder, sometimes the Box is contradictory. For example, one element of the "real man" myth is that a "real man" works with his hands. Another is that he runs the company and makes big money. So a mechanic might feel he's not a "real man" because he's not in big business. And a CEO might feel he's not a "real man" because he doesn't work with his hands.

The Box Leads Men to Be Inauthentic

Because it can be scary to be seen as "not a real man" and to catch the judgment and shaming that comes with that, one of the ways men often respond to situations in which they aren't fulfilling the expectations the Box creates is to act the role in the hope that no one will notice. This is why Kivel calls it the "Act Like a Man" Box. Sometimes men "perform" masculinity to avoid the harassment that men sometimes get when they aren't in the Box.

Unfortunately, this sometimes means not being true to oneself. A lot of men hide their feelings, since emotions other than anger are outside the Box, which often means they don't develop the ability to talk about how they feel. Other men might be interested in something other than sports, cars, and drinking with their buddies but either never try it or hide it from prying eyes. How guys dress, talk, work, and play is influenced by their perception that if they don't follow the rules, people will know that they aren't "real men." They may behave a certain way not because it is what they really want, but because they feel that they have something to prove.

The Box Values Performance over Pleasure

What do you suppose would happen if men had the choice between an 8-inch cock with limited sensation and a 4-inch cock with added sensation? We're pretty certain that some men would opt for less sensation if it meant having a bigger cock, and therefore being more "manly."

When you're stuck in the Box, fulfilling the expectations of being a "real man" is more important than experiencing pleasure, and sex is all about scoring and proving that you're macho. It becomes more important that a man should "perform" well than that he should enjoy himself. And if he's having sex with a woman, her enjoyment and her orgasms are sometimes not for her sake so much as a way to prove how good he is at what he's doing.

In the Box, it's all about the cock and what you do with it: "get it up, get it in, get it off." This is so central that some people have the expectation that men should get all their sexual pleasure from their penis, to the exclusion of the rest of their body. Despite the fact that men have sensitive spots all over, there's still a widespread belief that the penis is the only thing to pay attention to. We've heard men say things like "My cock is all I need to get off," as if it would be an offense to the sovereignty of the cock if other parts of his body added to his pleasure!

Plenty of men get stuck trying to fit themselves into a sexual script that might not always feel right to them. There's no limit to the ways in which we can have sex, and when you restrict yourself to the kinds of sex that fit into the Box, you miss out on a lot of amazing fun.

While we respect everyone's right and ability to enjoy whatever sexual pleasure they wish—within the bounds of the consent and well-being of everyone involved—we've noticed that there's a big difference between "I tried it and didn't like it" and the more defensive "I'll never do that." Unfortunately, it means that a lot of men choose the Box over their own pleasure.

PICKING AND CHOOSING FROM THE BOX

Many men find, with time and consideration, that while some elements of the Box may fit who they are, others do not, and they realize that they resent having these expectations put upon them. But how to get free of it?

A lot of people think that in order to get rid of the Box a man needs to reject *all* those expectations and be none of the things the Box requires a man to be. However, by doing this he gets out of one box and right back into another: the Anti-Box. You might know some of these guys—they don't allow themselves to feel or express anger, they don't ever speak up for what they want, and they tend to be pretty passive. Before, they felt they had to be everything that the Box is, and now they feel they have to be nothing that the Box is. They're still in a box, it's just the opposite box!

Instead, we think the way to get free of the Box is to reject the either/or-ness of it: let go of the idea that you have to be all or none. You can pick and choose! You can be some of the things in the Box—you don't have to be *all* of them.

This also means that you can start creating your own definition of what it means to be a man. You don't have to try to meet the expectations of the Box. Ultimately, your sense of value as a person—no matter where you fall on the gender spectrum—comes from within you. No one can give it to you—you have to find it within yourself. And no one can take it away either—it's always available inside you, even if you lose contact with it at times.

As you free yourself from the Box, consider whether you are spending time with people who are really stuck in the Box mentality—friends, co-workers, family members, romantic partners, and playmates. If there are people in your life who try to force you into this box, or any box, maybe they aren't people you want to spend so much time around. Also, it's important to ask yourself how much of this judgment might actually be coming from within you. Have you internalized these messages?

BACK TO PROSTATE PLAY

Now that we've talked about the Box and how masculinity standards are created and reinforced, let's go back to the three main pillars of the idea that receiving penetration will make you less of a man and see how it all ties in together.

Remember the names that men sometimes get called when they don't meet all the requirements of the Box? You may have noticed that they all fall into three categories: you're female, gay, or a loser. Some terms even carry connotations of more than one category. Consider, for instance, that the word *fag* connotes both gay and feminine, and the term *sissy* connotes both feminine and weak. The insulting associations between femininity and male homosexuality are so deeply intertwined that it's sometimes difficult to even distinguish between them.

We think this says some interesting things about how the Box defines both women and gay men. A big part of how people define what it means to be a "real man" is by putting down women and gay men, and by viewing the world in terms of dominance and submission or win–lose. In many ways, sexism and homophobia are the bricks that make up the Box and shame is the mortar that holds them together.

"Penetration is the woman's role"

Receiving penetration is sometimes thought of as the woman's role in sex. And since a big part of being a "real man" means that you don't do anything womanly, then of course receiving penetration doesn't fit. Some men fear that if they get penetrated, they are being feminized—turned into a sissy.

Of course, the negative judgment about a man taking on the woman's role only works if you think there's something wrong with being a woman. Many men have internalized this judgment without ever considering that it is based on the idea that women are inferior and therefore men should not be like them. Ask yourself: do you really believe that women are inferior? What's so wrong with women that it should be a terrible thing for men to resemble them?

Also, the idea that in sex men have one role and women have another is very restrictive. "Men should do all the giving and women should do all the receiving"—these roles work fine if your sex life consists only of fucking with the man controlling all the motion. But a lot of people with very satisfying sex lives have roles that are more blurred: for example, sometimes the woman hops on top and controls the motion, or fucks back on him from underneath. Sometimes the woman gives a blow job while the man sits back and receives. Who is playing what role then? It's not always an either/or.

It's also worth thinking about how it can still be a woman's role if a man is doing it. In some ways, it's similar to how women used to be attacked for wearing pants (i.e., "men's clothes"). In our view, if a woman is wearing pants, they're a woman's clothes. Similarly, if a man gets penetrated, it's *his* hot sex!

The belief that only certain people ever enjoy or engage in a particular sexual practice holds a lot of people back from trying something they might enjoy. We'd much rather have people decide what they want to do based on their (and their partner's) consent, pleasure, and well-being than on someone else's opinion of what they should do.

"Only gay men like to be penetrated"

Two popular myths are: 1) All gay men like to take it up the ass, and 2) Only gay men do this. These myths gave birth to another: Any man who wants to be penetrated must secretly be gay. Or even that being penetrated will actually make you gay!

This is one of those things that's more about perception than reality. Lots of heterosexual men enjoy anal play. After all, it's not as if gay and bi men are born with extra parts that straight guys don't have! There are responsive nerves that will work for you whether you are doing this with a man, a woman, or by yourself.

While we're willing to bet that the percentage of straight men who enjoy penetration is smaller than the percentage of gay men, that's likely to be because gay men are generally more open to the idea of it since it is discussed more openly, and because they have probably had at least a few experiences with a partner who knew how to do it and what it was like. But this simply means that lots of straight guys haven't had the chance to try it out! It's also worth noting that recent research has shown that when men sleep with other men, anal sex is not always so pivotal as many people think: many men who sleep with men actually don't like to be anally penetrated, and their play focuses on other acts such as blow jobs.

The important thing to know is that *whether* you like anal penetration is about what kinds of sexual stimulation work for you; *who* you want to do it with is about your sexual orientation. While there can be some correlation between the two, one doesn't imply anything about the other. If you're gay and you don't like anal play, you're still gay. If you're straight (or bi or any other sexual orientation) and you enjoy it, that doesn't make you gay.

And just to be clear, in our view, there's nothing wrong with any sexual orientation. But while we're on the subject,

> *"Do you have toys that are made for men?"*
>
> *"Yes. We have cock rings, sleeves, and anal toys—"*
>
> *"Do you have toys that are made for straight men?"*
>
> *"Yes. We have cock rings, sleeves, and anal toys."*
>
> —CONVERSATION WITH A MALE SHOPPER AT GOOD VIBRATIONS

we'd like to point out that the idea that a straight guy is less of a man if he takes it up the ass, because that's a gay thing to do, is based on homophobia, in the same way that concerns about assuming the woman's role stem from sexism. To get out of the Box and be able to fully enjoy yourself and your prostate explorations, you may have to root out absorbed views like this that you may not agree with!

"Penetration is an act of dominance"

The idea that being penetrated is a bad thing shows up in some interesting ways. For example, if you are in trouble, some people will say "You're fucked!" or "You're screwed!" The idea that penetration is an act of dominance is almost certainly tied in to sexism and the notion that the woman's role is inferior. Plenty of men have absorbed these ideas at a subconscious level. Even if a man doesn't think it is an act of dominance when he penetrates his (male or female) partner, he may still hesitate to switch roles because he is afraid that it will mean losing his masculinity if he takes a turn catching instead of pitching.

Certainly, penetration can be done in a spirit of dominance, but it isn't true that penetration is *always* an act of dominance. And just because it is sometimes viewed or performed that way doesn't mean it has to happen like that between you and your partner. It's all about how you do it, rather than anything inherent in the act of penetration.

First, let's investigate this idea of domination. What does it mean for one partner to dominate the other? As typically understood, it means that the dominant partner imposes their will on the other, who submits even if it's not what they want. Notice how this poses sex as a win–lose activity, where there can only be one winner and the other person loses. Let's not forget that many of the terms for men who don't fit inside the Box carry connotations of losing or submitting: *loser, weak, wimp, punk, bitch.*

It's not surprising that this polarity comes up around anal penetration, because there's a common myth that anal play always hurts the receiver and only feels good for the giver, and the receiver only does it because the giver wants it. We suspect this is also why some straight guys may fear that their female partners want to penetrate them not for mutual pleasure, but as some kind of passive-aggressive payback.

Of course, we know that this is not true: receiving penetration can actually feel really, really good—and often the receptive partner is the one who suggests it! How can they be losing when they are getting exactly what they want?

Instead of the win–lose mentality, where one person is dominant and the other person submits, we propose that sex can be a total win–win, where both the receiver and the giver: a) want to do it, b) enjoy it, and c) want their partner to enjoy it just as much.

> "When we moved to strap-on anal sex with him as the receptive partner, we were careful at first to be certain that neither of us saw this as an act of dominance. Satisfied that we did not see his penetrating my vagina as an act of dominance, we proceeded with hedonistic abandon."

Now that we've dispelled the myth that penetration is inherently an act of domination, we'd like to talk about fantasies. Many people are turned on by thinking about or acting out a situation of dominance and submission or force/coercion in sex. Doing this in your sex life is not the same as wanting it to happen in real life: you can enjoy these fantasies while being perfectly clear that you would never want to force someone or be forced in actuality.

Along those lines, some people enjoy settling into a submissive frame of mind when they get penetrated, as part of a mutually agreed upon BDSM role play. For them it's just a fantasy, and both partners are clear that it doesn't say anything about their real-life relationship. It's like a hat that you put on for a while and you can take off anytime.

If fantasies of dominance and submission (D/s) are a turn-on for you and your partner and you'd like to incorporate that into your prostate play, by all means go right ahead! (Just be sure to establish a safeword.) Violet Blue's book *The Ultimate Guide to Sexual Fantasy* has lots of great tips for exploring fantasies.

And, if you're not into that, then you don't have to go there. It's possible to enjoy prostate play without having any of those feelings at all.

When you start experimenting with prostate play, if you notice that the issue of dominance is getting in the way of enjoying yourself, take a break from doing it with a partner and spend some time with solo exploration. Going solo is a great way to set aside any partner expectations or concerns about how the play might affect your relationship and find out what you enjoy before bringing another person into the mix. It will let you explore the physical sensations of prostate play at your leisure, without the complications of attending to a partner.

IT'S UP TO YOU

Whether or not you would like to explore your prostate is up to you. Ultimately, we respect each person's ability to make this choice. But if you think that being penetrated makes a man less of a man, take some time to explore why you're letting that get in the way of enjoying yourself. There are many ways to be a man, and prostate play fits right into that for a lot of men.

Plenty of men—and lots of women—don't enjoy being penetrated for any of a number of reasons. The difference is between choosing not to do something because it doesn't feel good and believing that you can't do something because a "real man" supposedly wouldn't. It's a question of whether your decision is based on what works for you or on externally defined rules that are imposed on you.

Don't be discouraged if you have these concerns relating to masculinity: a lot of newbies to prostate play have to sort through these concerns before they can relax and enjoy themselves. Ironically, this also means (at least in our experience) that many of the men who get into anal penetration are among the most secure in their masculinity: because they've examined themselves, faced their fears, and worked through it.

We hope that you can find a definition of masculinity that

opens doors for you rather than closing them. Our hope is that however you choose to define your masculinity, you can find ways to enjoy the many pleasures that sex can bring, including prostate play.

PROSTATE HEALTH

Prostate conditions are fairly common. It's been said that "if you live a normal male lifespan, odds are at some point you will experience a prostate problem."[23] Some of these health concerns are more annoying than dangerous, while others can pose a serious threat. Fortunately, the best tool you have to maintain your prostate health is information, so read on for a description of the most common prostate conditions and what you can do about them.

PROSTATITIS

Prostatitis is a class of diseases with four types. We will describe the three most commonly diagnosed categories.

The literal meaning of the term *prostatitis* is "inflammation of the prostate." In its simplest form, prostatitis is an infection of the prostate by a microorganism that has traveled up the urethra and into the microscopic ducts and glands of the prostate. This is called Type I: acute bacterial prostatitis. There is a sudden onset of symptoms including pain in the prostate/perineum/lower back, pain and difficulty with urination, plus fever and chills. This form of prostatitis is the easiest to diagnose and treat. Signs of inflammation are found in the prostatic fluid and, if a culture is done, bacteria (or other likely-culprit microorganisms) are found as well. Most of the time, a complete course of antibiotics resolves the infection.

For some men, prostate infections become chronic. Many of the symptoms are the same, notably frequent and painful urination. But instead of coming on suddenly with fever and chills, symptoms appear gradually and ebb and flow over time, with periodic flare-ups. This is called Type II: chronic bacterial prostatitis. This most often occurs when a case of Type I: acute bacterial prostatitis is not fully cured and comes back. It can also occur in cases of recurrent urethral infection, or in patients with a history of repeated use of urethral instruments, such as sounds and catheters. There is inflammation and bacteria in the prostatic fluid, yet unlike Type I, the condition is not consistently cured by antibiotics. Doctors do not know why the antibiotics are sometimes ineffective. In some cases, multiple rounds of cultures and different types of antibiotics may clear the infection, but when that doesn't work, the prostate lives in a chronic state of inflammation.

A third category of prostatitis is even more trying. It is the most commonly diagnosed form of prostatitis, and also the hardest to cure—Type III: chronic pelvic pain syndrome. In this type, the patient has the usual pelvic pain and urinary symptoms, and occasionally sexual symptoms such as pain during ejaculation. In some cases, inflammation of the prostate is detected by finding inflammatory products (a nice way of saying pus) in the prostatic fluid or urine. In others, signs of inflammation are not found; inflammation may still be present but is not detected. Either way, no bacteria are found, and the cause of symptoms is unclear.

Cases such as these have historically been diagnosed as "nonbacterial prostatitis" because the symptoms are so similar to those of chronic bacterial prostatitis (Type II). This is so even though it is not clear that the prostate is the origin of symptoms in Type III cases. In this way, the term *prostatitis* became, in the words of one urologist, "a wastebasket of clinical ignorance, used to describe any condition associated with prostatic inflammation or prostatic symptoms."[24] It has been suggested that the syndromes which are lumped into the category of "prostatitis" may actually be several different diseases with similar symptoms.[25]

In 1995, the National Institutes of Health (NIH) held a convention to redefine the categories of prostatitis. They pointed out that in some cases of prostatitis the cause was unknown and that "organs other than the prostate gland may be involved." It was at this point that the category of "nonbacterial prostatitis" was replaced by the new category Type III: chronic pelvic pain syndrome (CPPS).[26]

Because prostatitis Types II and III are so similar in their chronic nature and the difficulty of treatment, they are often referred to collectively as CP/CPPS. To the frustration of doctors and patients alike, many men struggle with these conditions on an ongoing basis. This is an active area of research, and many studies are currently under way to fill in the many unknowns.

NATIONAL INSTITUTES OF HEALTH CATEGORIES OF PROSTATITIS

Type I: acute bacterial prostatitis. Bacterial infection of the prostate with sudden onset, fever and chills. Bacteria are detected, usually cured by antibiotics if full dose is taken.

Type II: chronic bacterial prostatitis. Ongoing or recurrent bacterial infection and inflammation of the prostate, often associated with frequent UTIs (urinary tract infections). Difficult to cure, even with antibiotics.

Type III: chronic pelvic pain syndrome (CPPS). There is pain, and sometimes inflammation, but no bacteria are found in cultures. Difficult to cure. Previously called chronic nonbacterial prostatitis or prostatodynia.

Type IV: asymptomatic inflammatory prostatitis. There are no symptoms, but bacteria or signs of inflammation are found in prostatic fluid during examination for other conditions.

WHAT IS INFLAMMATION?

Inflammation is a major symptom of Type I and II prostatitis, and it occurs in some cases of Type III. Even in cases of Type III where signs of inflammation are not found, it may still be present and undetected. Inflammation is the immune system's response to a perceived threat or injury: white blood cells are sent to the area to kill germs and do away with dead cells and irritants. In the case of prostatitis, inflammation is detected by looking at prostatic fluid or a urine sample through a microscope to check for a high number of white blood cells. Inflammation is not the same thing as infection: in an infection, microbes are present, while inflammation is the body's protective response to microbes, injury, irritation, or other harmful stimuli.

Usually, inflammation stops when the threat has been dealt with and the damage healed. However, sometimes it becomes chronic, and the inflammatory process happens on an ongoing basis. This changes the tissue environment and may even cause damage. Inflammation has been established as playing a role in a number of cancers,[27] and recent studies suggest that it may play a role in the development of prostate cancer and BPH.[28]

What Causes Prostatitis?

With Type I: acute prostatitis, the cause is clear—a bacterial infection, which clears up with antibiotics. Simple. With Types II and III (CP/CPPS), it's not so simple. If Type II is caused by infection, why don't antibiotics always work? And if the infection is not really the cause of symptoms, what is? What causes the symptoms of CPPS, given that no microorganisms are detected in cultures? These questions are unresolved, though there are many theories. Here are some of them.

Blocked glands may trap prostatic fluid and prevent it from being flushed out with ejaculation, forming a cozy breeding ground for bacteria. It may be that a microorganism is undetectable, has evolved immunity to antimicrobials, or is protected by a biofilm within the prostate. (A biofilm is a protective casing created by microorganisms such as bacteria. Plaque on your teeth is an example of a biofilm. It has been suggested that antibiotics do not work in some chronic infections because they cannot get through the biofilm to the microorganisms inside.)

If symptoms are not related to infection, other factors have been suggested, including urinary backflow, prostate stones, or other irritants in the gland. Any of these could potentially cause inflammation in the absence of microorganisms. Yet another possibility is that inflammation may occur in the absence of bacteria as a result of an overactive immune system, in which the immune response continues even after any threat or damage is eliminated.

One recent and promising theory is that, in at least some cases, the cause is muscle tension. The authors of *A Headache in the Pelvis* note that many men who have been diagnosed with CP/CPPS also have chronic tension in the muscles of the pelvis. The authors suggest that in some cases, CP/CPPS may arise as a result of this chronic tension. Some people tighten their pelvic muscles during anxiety—this is part of a natural instinct to protect the lower abdominal contents by tightening the muscles around them. The authors explain how, over time, this may lead to a vicious circle: anxiety causes tightening, which causes pain, which causes more anxiety, and so on.

The authors suggest that, over the course of many years of habitual tightening, the pelvic muscles may become shortened and chronically tense, which may interfere with the proper functioning of the nerves and blood vessels in the area. They suggest that this may be the original cause in many cases of CP/CPPS, and may even increase a man's likelihood of contracting Type I: acute prostatitis. In support of their theory, they have achieved good results in treating men with CP/CPPS: through physical therapy (myofascial release and relaxation training) they have been able to significantly reduce or eliminate symptoms in many men. (See the Resources for more information.)

PROSTATE HEALTH TIPS

There are many things you can do to support prostate health. We discuss a few here.

Keep the Urethra Healthy

Urethral health is important to prostate health. Since the urethra runs through the middle of the prostate, it is possible for an infectious agent to travel up the urethra and enter the ducts and glands of the prostate, causing an infection (acute prostatitis). The chances of this happening are increased if a urinary tract infection (UTI) is left untreated. Symptoms of a UTI include burning and pain when you pee and having to go more often than usual. If you have these symptoms, see a doctor. If antibiotics are prescribed, be sure to take the full course. Do not stop early even if the symptoms clear up; there may still be a low-level infection present that could make a comeback.

Avoid touching your urethral opening if your hands are not clean. Risk factors for UTI include catheters and urethral sounds. If you have a catheter or sound inserted (for medical reasons or in the context of kinky play) be sure to drink lots of fluids afterward to flush out the urethra. Don't start and stop the flow of urine; this may cause reflux urine to wash back into the prostate, causing irritation.[29]

Wear a Condom

Being on the giving end of unprotected sex increases your risk of contracting a UTI because you are exposing the opening of the urethra to any bacteria that are present. This is particularly true for unprotected anal sex, since the rectum contains a very wide range of microorganisms. For this reason, having unprotected anal sex as the giver, with a partner of any gender, is considered a risk factor for prostatitis.[30] Wearing a condom reduces this risk.

Pee after Sex

If you have sex without a condom, urinating afterward helps flush out the urethra. Drinking lots of water will help too.

Eat for Prostate Health

Studies increasingly indicate that diet and lifestyle have an impact on prostate health. Some studies suggest that particular nutrients may be linked to lower rates of prostate disease, and there are several prostate health cookbooks full of recipes that include these nutrients.

Not everyone feels that these diets are necessary. We

checked with Dr. Alan Shindel, assistant professor of urology at UC Davis, on the subject. He said, "Across the board, the diet that has been shown to be best for the health of every part of the body is whatever is smart for the heart. So a prudent diet (fruits, veggies, whole grains, light on the fats and fried foods) is best according to our knowledge."

That being said, most of the recipes in a prostate diet cookbook will be both heart-healthy and selected for nutrients that support prostate health, so if you feel inspired to try them, go right ahead!

Herbal Supplements

Many herbal supplements may also support prostate health. For a guide to herbal supplements, consult *Dr. Katz's Guide to Prostate Health: From Conventional to Holistic Therapies.*

BENIGN PROSTATIC HYPERPLASIA (BPH)

Benign prostatic hyperplasia (BPH) is overgrowth of the prostate. It is sometimes called "benign prostatic hypertrophy," but this is a misnomer. Hypertrophy means that cells of the body are growing in size, but in BPH the growth happens as a result of cells increasing in number. The term *benign* is used to differentiate this condition from cancerous growth. In the case of BPH, it is not cancer cells that are multiplying, so it is not life-threatening.

BPH usually occurs in the area of the prostate that immediately surrounds the urethra. This can make urination difficult if the growth of the prostate pinches off or blocks the urethra. Symptoms of BPH include difficulty starting the flow of urine, weak flow, frequent urge to go (especially at night), and feeling like the bladder is not empty even after going. The bladder muscles are working against the resistance of the prostate, and over time this muscular strain may cause the bladder muscles to become weak. This can lead to incomplete emptying of the bladder and, as a result, an increased likelihood of bladder infection.

The cause of BPH is not known, but age is a factor: most of the men who have symptoms are over age 50,[31] and your chances of developing the condition increase the older you get. The prostate undergoes growth at particular points in a man's life. In a boy the prostate is very small and underdeveloped. Then, at the start of puberty, there is a growth spurt. A second growth spurt comes in the mid-20s, and this growth continues (very slowly) throughout his life.[32] This is why BPH is so common among older men, and why their prostate may feel less regular, larger than average, and have less clearly defined lobes. All men experience some prostate growth as they age, but not all men will have the kind of growth that leads to urine obstruction and BPH symptoms.

The most common treatment for BPH symptoms is alpha blockers or 5-alpha reductase inhibitors. If these don't work or the patient cannot tolerate them, the doctor may recommend surgical intervention: transurethral resection of the prostate (TURP). This involves inserting a device into the urethra and surgically removing a small portion of the prostate to relieve the pressure on the urethra. Retrograde ejaculation is typical after this procedure. This is likely due to damage to the sphincter muscle that lies between the prostate and bladder, which pinches off the urethra during ejaculation to keep semen from entering the bladder. If this sphincter is damaged, semen may flow up into the bladder during ejaculation instead of out through the penis. The next time he urinates, it'll simply get flushed out. His urine will be cloudy, but there's no known health risk from it. Reduced semen volume may also result from removal of some of the glandular tissue of the prostate during TURP, which means less prostatic fluid is being produced in the first place. Some men also report a difference in the sensation experienced at orgasm after TURP. Long-term impotence or incontinence occurs in a small percentage of cases.[33]

PROSTATE CANCER

According to the American Cancer Society's 2010 estimates, 1 out of 6 men in the United States will be diagnosed with prostate cancer at some point in their lives, and 1 out of 36 men will die of the disease.

What Is Cancer, Anyway?

The life cycle of a cell includes a process called *apoptosis*— the programmed death of the cell. Apoptosis allows old cells to be broken down, recycled into the body, and replaced by healthy new cells. Cancer develops when changes in cellular DNA result in the cell's failure to go through apoptosis and die when its time comes. Instead, cancer cells live abnormally long lives. Cell division continues, thereby creating more and more cancer cells. As the population of cancer cells increases, they may form a detectable lump: a tumor. Eventually, the increasing number of cancer cells can interfere with the proper functioning of the affected body part. Worse yet, cancer cells sometimes travel to other sites: this is called metastasis. Once they settle in another part of the body, they continue to multiply in the new area.

Symptoms of Prostate Cancer

Prostate cancer would be much less troublesome if it were not for metastasis—the process by which cancer cells migrate to other parts of the body. Cancer cells within the prostate gland don't cause much trouble. The prostate is not a vital organ—you can survive just fine without it (though you might miss having it massaged). What causes life-threatening health problems is the spread of cancer cells to more vital parts of your body where they interfere with crucial life processes.

This is why prostate cancer is so markedly symptom-free. Most cases of prostate cancer are diagnosed in a total absence of symptoms. When symptoms do occur, they may include:

- Frequent or urgent need to urinate, difficulty in passing urine, interrupted or weakened flow of urine, dribbling afterward

- Pain during urination or ejaculation

- Blood in the urine or semen

- Pain or stiffness in the lower back, pelvis, hips, or thighs

- Partial erections or impotence

- Decreased quantity of semen during ejaculation

However, by the time these symptoms occur, the cancer is usually very advanced and may already have spread (metastasized) to other parts of the body where it poses a much more serious threat. This is why some doctors recommend screening for early detection. However, there is some controversy about the value of screening and aggressive treatment of prostate cancers. We discuss this a little later.

Causes and Risk Factors

Modern science has not yet discovered the cause of prostate cancer, though it is speculated that hormones play a role. In cases of very advanced prostate cancer, reducing the man's testosterone level slows the growth of the cancer. This has led many to believe that testosterone feeds prostate cancer growth and to caution against the use of chemical testosterone, which is sometimes prescribed to men with low testosterone levels.

However, this has recently come into question. Ernani Luis Rhoden MD and Abraham Morgentaler MD published a study in which they state, "Despite decades of research, there is no compelling evidence that testosterone has a causative role in prostate cancer." They point out that just because cutting off testosterone slows cancer growth does not necessarily mean that increasing testosterone will promote growth. Further, many men with low testosterone levels have prostate cancer, and since testosterone levels tend to decrease with age, "prostate cancer becomes more prevalent exactly at the time of a man's life when testosterone levels decline."[34]

Lately, also, a great deal of attention has been given to the fact that many cancers, including prostate cancer, grow in an environment of chronic inflammation such as occurs with prostatitis. Some studies suggest that inflammation may play a causative role in the development of cancer.

There are several risk factors for prostate cancer. Notably, older men are at a much higher risk, starting around age 50. From there, the risk increases with the years, and approximately two-thirds of cases are diagnosed in men over 65.[35] If you have relatives with prostate cancer, you are at high risk for developing it. Furthermore, if your relatives were diagnosed at a relatively young age (before 50), you are at an increased risk of having it while young. Race is relevant as well: African American men living in the US are more at risk than any other racial group, and more likely to die from it. The reason for this is uncertain, but research is under way to answer this and other questions related to prostate cancer.

Other possible risk factors include nationality/geography (some countries have higher rates than others) and diet.

Screening for Prostate Cancer

As mentioned, prostate cancer is generally asymptomatic until the disease is very advanced, so it is usually diagnosed through routine screening. However, there is some controversy over the value of screening. (See the section "The Screening Controversy" that begins on page 291.) The American Cancer Society recommends that men discuss screening options with their doctor and make an informed decision about whether or not to pursue it. They recommend that this conversation take place at age 50 for men with average risk, age 45 for men with high risk (African American men or men with a close relative who was diagnosed at an early age), and age 40 for men with multiple close relatives who were diagnosed at an early age.[36]

Two tests are commonly used to screen for prostate cancer. First is the digital rectal exam (DRE)—a finger exam. (Before computers, the word *digital* referred to fingers.) The doctor inserts a gloved, lubricated finger into the rectum and manually checks the surface of the prostate for lumps which may be cancerous tumors.

Second is the PSA test. PSA stands for *prostate specific antigen*, a protein that is released by the prostate. The test monitors the level of PSA in your bloodstream. Levels vary from person to person and over time, so when the doctor checks your PSA, he is less interested in the actual level of your PSA on a given day than in the rate of change over time. He is watching for sharp increases, which could indicate cancer.

Studies suggest that ejaculation[37] and prostate massage[38] may cause a temporary increase in your PSA level, which could raise a red flag on your test. For this reason, some doctors recommend that you abstain from all sexual activity for at least 48 hours before the test.

PROSTATE CANCER SCREENING FOR TRANSGENDER WOMEN

At present, most sex realignment surgery for transgender women leaves the prostate intact, placing it in the location where the G-spot would be in relation to the neovagina. This allows transgender women to keep a very erotically responsive tissue and adds to the pleasure they can experience with intercourse. It also means that they are still at risk for prostate cancer.

Some have speculated that transgender women who take feminizing hormones (antiandrogens) have a reduced risk of developing a fatal case of prostate cancer. This is believed to be the case because blocking a cisgender man's testosterone in cases of advanced prostate cancer has been shown to slow the growth of the cancer. The antiandrogens that are prescribed to these men are some of the same ones prescribed to transgender women to block testosterone and other androgens in order to feminize the body. So some have suggested that the antiandrogens would have the same effect in transgender women as they have in advanced cases of prostate cancer in cisgender men: to slow the development of any prostate cancer that may be present.

It's important to note that this has not been proven. Transgender health is a very young field of research and very little is known so far. Even if it is true that antiandrogens might slow the development of a prostate cancer, it doesn't halt it entirely, so there is still a risk there. Also, as Alan Shindel points out, "There are published studies indicating that cisgender males with low testosterone are still at risk for aggressive prostate cancers," so a low testosterone level is no guarantee.

Since there is still a risk, transgender women who are in the screening age range may choose to see a urologist for annual prostate screening. (Likewise, many doctors recommended that female-to-male transgender men see a gynecologist for cervical cancer screening.)

It may be scary for a transgender woman to go to a doctor's

office where she may expect that all other patients will be men. However, unlike gynecologists, who do not see cisgender men, urologists see both men and women. A cisgender woman may visit a urologist for a urinary system issue such as incontinence, urinary stones, or cancers of the urinary system organs, so while there may be fewer women in the waiting room than men, it's not unusual for a woman to see a urologist.

Still, transgender women may have concerns about whether the particular urologist will be open to seeing a transgender person and will treat them with the same respect as anyone else. If you are concerned about how you will be received, call the office, tell them your situation, and ask them frankly if they are comfortable seeing you. If they fumble over the phone, it saves you the hassle of going in.

There are more transgender-friendly doctors than ever before, so look for one in your area. Ask around among queer/trans-aware people or contact local LGBTQ organizations for a recommendation. Also, see the Resources for a link to a database of LGBTQ-friendly health professionals.

The Screening Controversy

Because prostate cancer rarely shows symptoms until it is too late to cure it, many doctors place a high emphasis on early screening and aggressive treatment of this disease. However, this has led to some controversy.

Relative to many other cancers, prostate cancer tends to grow slowly, and may exist in the prostate for years without decreasing quality of life. There have even been cases where men have died of an unrelated cause and were found, during autopsy, to have had a slow-growing tumor in the prostate.

In these cases, if the men had been diagnosed with cancer and had gone through all the stress, pain, financial burden, and decreased quality of life that comes with treatment, they would have done so unnecessarily, since the cancer never would have caused trouble during their lifetime.

This creates a dilemma for medical professionals: how vigorously should prostate cancer be screened, diagnosed, and treated given that in some cases the cancer may never cause any problems and the patient may die without ever knowing he had it? Or worse—given that in some cases the treatment for prostate cancer may actually cause more suffering than the cancer itself would have? (Incidentally, this is why urologists don't do prostate cancer screening for men with a life expectancy of less than 10 years.)

Recently, the U.S. Preventive Services Task Force actually recommended *against* the use of the PSA test in screening. Its reasoning was that, first, studies suggest that early detection of prostate cancer may not actually extend the lives of patients. And second, since the test can't tell between life-threatening cancers and slow-growing cancers, it may do more harm than good, as mentioned above, by causing anxiety, pain, financial burden, and decreased quality of life to many men with manageable cancers.

Because screening has become controversial, many medical professionals recommend that men talk with their doctors about the possible benefits of screening and decide for themselves whether they will pursue it. To be clear, some men do die of prostate cancer, so screening may be of benefit to some men.

Treatment

If prostate cancer is found early, the patient may choose not to pursue any treatment right away. Since many cases of prostate cancer are very slow growing, the patient may enjoy years of uninterrupted quality of life and postpone more aggressive treatment until it is necessary. This is called watchful waiting, or active surveillance, where the patient collaborates with the doctor to monitor the development of the cancer over time. Typically, it involves regularly scheduled visits for blood tests and DRE exams, and perhaps repeated biopsies of the prostate. Some use the terms *watchful waiting* and *active surveillance* interchangeably, while others consider them to be different, active surveillance referring to a more aggressive approach than watchful waiting.

When the patient decides to pursue treatment to eliminate the cancer, and if the cancer has not grown beyond the capsule of the prostate, the most common procedure is radical prostatectomy—the surgical removal of the gland. Another form of treatment is radiation therapy, either by way of external beam radiation or radioactive "seeds" that are implanted into the prostate. Numerous other forms of treatment are also being researched.

If the cancer has spread to lymph nodes, bone, or other organs, it cannot be cured, and the focus of treatment shifts to slowing its growth and minimizing symptoms.

SEX AFTER PROSTATE CANCER TREATMENT
Erectile Function

It used to be that surgical removal of the prostate meant complete loss of erectile function, leading to the common jest that the cure for prostate cancer is worse than the disease. The reason why removal of the prostate interferes with erectile function has to do with two bundles of nerves that flank the prostate on each side. These nerves play an important role in erection, and they run alongside the prostate on their way to the penis, so they are easily damaged during prostate removal.

Previously, doctors were not aware of the role that these nerves played in a man's ability to get hard, so they would take them out along with the prostate, resulting in a high rate of erectile dysfunction. Today many doctors practice a "nerve sparing" technique: whenever possible they leave one or both of these nerve bundles in place. Of course, this isn't always possible. If it appears that the cancer has moved beyond the prostate, the doctor may choose to remove some surrounding tissue in an effort to ensure that all cancer cells have been eliminated. This may mean taking out the nerve segments along with the affected tissue.

When one or both nerves are spared, erectile function can usually recover beginning at two to three months and increasing for up to two years following surgery. This means that erection rates post-surgery are much better than they used to be before nerve-sparing techniques were developed.

However, even among men who regain erectile function after surgery, it may not be what it once was. Along these lines, whether or not an erection functions may vary by sex act. A super-hard erection is not required for vaginal sex, but it usually takes a pretty solid erection for anal penetration, since the anus tends to be tighter than the vaginal opening. Jerry Harris, a contributing author of *A Gay Man's Guide to Prostate Cancer*, notes that in his experience many gay men are bottoms after prostate removal, even in some cases where they were tops beforehand. Point being: the question of whether or not your post-surgery erection functions depends in part on what you want to do with it.

Men who have consistent erections before the surgery have a better chance of regaining erectile function afterward. It's a prime example of "use it or lose it": you have a better chance of regaining and maintaining your erectile function after the procedure if you keep up an active (solo or partnered) sex life. Also, many doctors recommend taking an erection drug like Viagra, Levitra, or Cialis on a regular basis after surgery in the hope that regular increases in blood flow will assist the recovery of erectile function; however, a recent study suggested that better results may be achieved by taking these pills on demand, as they are needed.[39]

Radiation therapy can also decrease erectile function.[40] In a reverse trend, with these procedures erectile function is initially unchanged, but may slowly decrease over time. At present, studies suggest that the procedure least damaging to erectile function is brachytherapy—radiation therapy that involves planting radioactive "seeds" or wires inside the prostate at the location of the tumor.[41] However, even though brachytherapy may cause the least impairment, all treatments for prostate cancer typically have a negative effect on sexual function.

The Prostate after Cancer

A lot of what is written about prostate cancer covers in detail the effects of treatment on erectile function, but very few articles mention the effect on receptive anal penetration or, for that matter, prostate pleasure. This is due to a lack of attention to these sexual practices by many medical professionals. Most information on sexual function after prostate cancer treatment focuses on heterosexual vaginal sex; there is little information on other types of couples or other types of sex.

At this time there are no studies on the effect that the various prostate cancer treatments have on prostate massage, though there are some reports from the experiences of individuals.

First, after surgical removal of the prostate, it's just gone: you will no longer be able to massage it. You can still enjoy anal penetration for its own sake; the nerves of the anus and rectum will still be receptive as they were before. Plenty of men continue to enjoy anal play after having their prostate removed. Unfortunately, if your prostate is a big part of what you enjoy about anal penetration, you'll probably experience a decrease in sensation.

It is unclear how radiation therapy affects prostate sensation. We have spoken with at least one man who still enjoyed prostate massage following external beam radiation therapy (radiation applied to the prostate in a beam from outside the body), though it is hard to say whether his pleasure was simply coming from the anal penetration and not the prostate massage. Furthermore, radiation works by killing the cells of the prostate, so it is likely that any remaining sensation will be greatly decreased.

It should also be noted that your ability to receive anal penetration may be affected by some forms of treatment. In external beam radiation therapy, mentioned above, some radiation may contact the rectum, causing irritation in the form of diarrhea, rectal bleeding, and discomfort and putting receptive anal penetration on hold. Usually the symptoms pass after treatment is completed. Occasionally the irritation persists, which may mean a permanent halt to anal sex. (This is rare.) If you choose the other form of radiation, brachytherapy (seed implanting), irritation of the rectum is less likely, though your doctor may recommend that you refrain from receiving anal sex for a period after implantation while the seeds are radioactive (about 6 weeks).[42]

Other Effects

Most men have dry orgasms after prostate cancer treatment: they don't ejaculate any fluid. A study on orgasm after radical prostatectomy indicated that for some men the lack of ejaculation diminishes their experience of pleasure at orgasm.[43] Also, those who eroticize semen may miss having it as a part of the experience. Generally, dry orgasm also means infertility.

Also of note, the length of the penis may decrease slightly after prostate removal. Some men also have issues with urinary continence (holding their urine) after prostate treatment. Stress incontinence is common after radical prostatectomy, and some men report an emission of urine with ejaculation.[44] Some men also experience urge incontinence after radiation therapy. Incontinence issues may improve over time, or they may be persistent. This can be very challenging—many people find loss of bladder control highly embarrassing. However, some men have eroticized this by getting into water sports!

POSSIBLE BENEFITS
OF PROSTATE MASSAGE

In 2008, an online advertisement for the Nexus line of prostate massagers featured a woman giving this enthusiastic endorsement: "Prostate massage isn't just for fun though, guys—it's also recommended by doctors as an aid to the prevention of prostate cancer." This may sound like an outlandish claim, but there is some evidence that prostate massage may be beneficial to the health of your prostate.

It is possible that regular, repeated massage helps prevent the development of some prostate diseases. At times, it has even been used in the treatment of prostate conditions. (We discuss this below.) While there are few studies on the subject that provide indisputable evidence, there are reasons to believe that prostate massage may be useful.

> # HAVE SYMPTOMS? SEE A DOCTOR
>
> If you have symptoms of a prostate disease, we recommend that you see a doctor. We are not medical doctors, and we do not present this information to diagnose any condition or recommend any form of treatment.
>
> Also, if you have symptoms of acute prostatitis (especially fever and chills—see chapter 14, Prostate Health) you should refrain from prostate massage. In addition to feeling terrible, massaging a prostate with an active infection may push bacteria into the bloodstream and promote sepsis (blood poisoning).

HOW MAY PROSTATE MASSAGE BE BENEFICIAL?

How, exactly, is prostate massage supposed to help keep your prostate healthy? There are a number of possible benefits of massage for general prostate health, sexual fitness, and some specific conditions. Here they are.

> *"The benefit from prostatic massage is believed to be derived from a combination of several factors, including expression of inspissated prostatic secretions, relief of pelvic muscle spasm, physical disruption of any protective biofilm, improved circulation, and consequently improved antibiotic penetration."*
>
> —VIBHASH C. MISHRA, JOHN BROWNE, AND MARK EMBERTON

Increasing Circulation

Massage of any part of the body helps to increase circulation of blood and lymph fluids in that area. Blood flow is important to the healthy functioning of cells and tissues because it brings fresh oxygen and nutrients that your body needs to run properly. Because prostate massage is so often arousing, you get the added increase of blood flow that comes with arousal. Arousal causes the whole pelvic area to engorge with blood, particularly after ejaculation. An ultrasound study has shown that blood flow to the prostate increases significantly after ejaculation and stays elevated for up to 24 hours afterward.[45]

If you have a chronic prostate infection (chronic prostatitis) and you are taking antibiotics, the increased blood flow from prostate massage may (theoretically) facilitate getting the medication in your bloodstream to the prostate. This means that prostate massage may make antibiotics more effective at clearing chronic prostate infections.

Releasing Muscle Tension

Massage in general can be very relaxing, and this is no less true for prostate massage, especially when easy, gentle penetration is used. Anal penetration requires a certain degree of muscle relaxation simply to allow the sphincters to open. Also, during penetration, a number of deep pelvic muscles may receive secondary massage and partake in the overall relaxation and openness of the area.

Having chronically tight muscles in the pelvis can reduce circulation and interfere with function. Recently, a group of researchers at Stanford University suggested that pelvic muscle tension may be a cause or contributing factor in many cases of CP/CPPS. Dr. David Wise and Dr. Rodney Anderson describe this theory in their book *A Headache in the Pelvis*. Over time, they say, "the state of chronic constriction creates pain-referring trigger points, reduced blood flow, and an inhospitable environment for the nerves, blood vessels, and structures throughout the pelvic basin."[46] They developed a protocol to treat CP/CPPS patients with relaxation training and myofascial release, with some noteworthy success. According to one study of 116 men with a median of 6 months of follow-up, 82 percent of the men reported symptom improvement.[47]

Certainly, your run-of-the mill prostate massage takes a much less exacting approach to muscular relaxation than the Wise-Anderson protocol. Nevertheless, prostate massage (and anal penetration generally) may bring about some muscle release by applying indirect pressure to tight pelvic muscles and inviting them to relax. Since chronically tight pelvic muscles can create an "inhospitable environment" for nerves and blood vessels, they can actually decrease the sensation that you can feel. So, if you practice prostate massage in a relaxing way, it can help support sexual functioning and pleasure by restoring tense muscles to a healthier, more relaxed state that will allow more circulation and more sensation.

Along these lines, many men report having harder erections after they begin exploring prostate massage, which may be due to relaxed pelvic muscles allowing greater blood flow to the penis. According to Daniel W. Nixon and Max Gomez, authors of *The Prostate Health Program: A Guide to Preventing and Controlling Prostate Cancer*, "Some sexual disorders, such as weak erections, premature ejaculation, and impotence, can benefit from prostatic massage or Kegel exercises."[48]

Flushing Out Fluids and Clearing Blockages

With prostate massage, accumulated prostatic fluid may be pushed out of the microscopic glands and into the urethra, where it will be flushed away with urination or ejaculation. This may help clear the prostate of fluid which contains potentially harmful matter such as pathogens and wastes remaining from the inflammatory process. In this way, regular prostate massage may theoretically reduce the risk of developing prostate conditions by flushing out harmful agents before they can do harm.

But wait—flushing out the fluids? Isn't that what happens during ejaculation? Yes, but some speculate that blockages in the ducts and glands can trap fluid, and these blocked glands may become breeding grounds for bacteria and centers of chronic inflammation. It is possible that ejaculation alone may not be strong enough to clear these blockages, but prostate massage may open them, at least temporarily, allowing the trapped fluid and any irritants it contains to drain out.

A few doctors who practice prostate massage as a treatment for prostatitis presented work to support this idea at the Third International Chronic Prostatitis Network conference in 2000. They collected semen samples and post-massage prostatic fluid from 10 men with symptoms of chronic prostatitis. When comparing the samples, they found that eight of the 10 men had signs of inflammation in the prostatic fluid, but not in the semen.

Based on this small sample, they suggested that in at least some prostatitis patients, regular ejaculation is not strong enough to clear all of the prostatic fluid from the gland, and may leave behind some fluid that contains inflammatory agents that can be forced out by prostate massage.[49] So it is possible that prostate massage may clear out more prostatic fluid than ejaculation alone.

Breaking Up Stones, Disrupting Biofilms

One possible reason why some cases of CP/CPPS do not respond to antibiotics is that there may be a bacterial biofilm. Biofilms are like bacteria cities in which the microbes produce a coating that encapsulates them and protects them from the environment, allowing them to survive an onslaught of antibiotics. Plaque is one example of a biofilm. If in some cases a biofilm in the prostate is responsible for CP/CPPS symptoms, it is speculated that massage could cause a physical disruption of the biofilm, allowing some antibiotics to get inside to the bacteria that are fortressed within.

Another cause of CP/CPPS symptoms may be the presence of prostatic stones—calcifications within the microscopic glands of the prostate. Some recommend vigorous massage to break up the stones, the fragments of which have been found in prostatic fluid following massage. If the stones are in fact contributing to symptoms, this may be of benefit, though some suggest that such aggressive massage may actually be traumatic to the prostate.

Greater Awareness of Prostate Health

Through prostate massage, you can become more aware of your prostate, more familiar with its normal state, and more capable of recognizing the onset of unusual symptoms. One man described how his familiarity with his prostate helped him when he came down with a prostate infection: "When I had a bacterial prostate infection, I could feel the swelling and the heat in my prostate. I knew that's where it was because I was familiar with my prostate from having done prostate play many times. So I was able to tell my doctor that's what it felt like, which she confirmed with an exam." Also, if your partner gives you prostate massages, he or she may be able to monitor your prostate over time and notice if there is a lump, which might indicate prostate cancer.

A LITTLE HISTORY

"For the treatment of the chronically diseased prostate, massage of that organ by the rectum, constitutes the most important element of the treatment."

—JAMES BAYARD CLARK (ON PROSTATITIS, WRITING IN 1912)

Prostate massage has a fascinating medical history. In the United States, it was a common form of treatment practiced by physicians between the late 1800s and the first two decades of the 1900s. In the words of one doctor from 1895, "'Milking the prostate,' and 'milking the seminal vesicles' [...] has recently become somewhat of a fad."[50]

If you look at medical books from this period, you can find detailed descriptions of how to perform prostate massage as a treatment for various ailments. Depending on the condition, the patient might see the doctor as often as daily for a brief massage. Frequently, treatment also included the use of urethral sounds and the insertion of a solution into the prostatic urethra.

Prostate massage was used for many conditions, but most commonly for treating prostatitis. This was before the dawn of antibiotics, and gonorrheal infections of the urethra frequently made their way into the prostate, causing prostatitis (Type I or Type II). The purpose of the massage was to support the lymphatic and circulatory systems, to desensitize an overly tender prostate, and to wring out the contents of the gland.[51]

Massage was also used for sexual disorders, including impotence. In 1912, one physician recommended prostate massage at the doctor's office one or two times weekly to treat impotence. He also suggested using a vibrator to massage the gland for three to five minutes every day.[52] At times, massage was also used for premature ejaculation,[53] priapism,[54] and "exaggerated libido."[55]

In addition to the use of prostate massage by doctors, there was a whole industry of "quacks" who favored this technique. These questionable practitioners without medical degrees placed ads in newspapers offering cures for various ailments, many of which were considered by most doctors to be of little consequence. Judging from the many references to "quacks" by doctors of the period, it seems that there was a booming industry of prostate massage for "imaginary ailments."[56]

MEDICAL HISTORY OF THE ANEROS

The medical use of prostate massage was the inspiration for the ever-popular Aneros prostate massager. Developed in the late 1990s, it was invented as a tool to allow men to perform prostate massage on themselves at home for health purposes. Named the "Pro-State Massager," it was designed and subsequently patented by Japanese urologist Dr. Jiro Takashima and manufactured through High Island Health, LLC.

As men tried the product, more and more of them reported some rather pleasant and unexpected side effects on their sex lives. The benefits they experienced were likely a result of both the prostate massage and the pelvic muscle strengthening that occurs when you use the Aneros in the hands-free way it was designed for, where you create the motion by flexing and releasing your pelvic muscles. (See chapter 11, Toys, for more information on the Aneros.) Once High Island Health, LLC, realized that the product was selling more as a sex toy than a health aid, it began to market it that way under the Aneros Company.[57]

The Hysteria Parallel

From as early as the 5th century BC there are references in Western medicine to a disease known (primarily) as "hysteria" that was thought to afflict women. It is no longer considered a legitimate diagnosis, but until fairly recent history it was believed to be a disease of the uterus that resulted from insufficient sexual gratification.

The treatment, which some women required repeatedly, was for a doctor or midwife to massage the woman's vulva to the point of "hysterical paroxysm" (an orgasm!).

This phenomenon is well documented in *The Technology of Orgasm,* by Rachel P. Maines. Hysteria diagnosis and treatment in the US peaked from the turn of the century to around 1920. In an interesting parallel, prostate massage also had its heyday as a medical treatment in the US during this period. In the same way that hysteria treatment involved the "hysterical paroxysm" (orgasm), much of the literature on prostate massage emphasizes the "relief" of prostate "congestion."[58] The phrase "milking the prostate" was often used, emphasizing the forcing out of secretions. In some cases this occurred "at once from the meatus."[59] This sounds a lot like ejaculation.

There were even some remarkable devices for physician-administered prostate massages. Just as the vibrator was, at the turn of the century, a new invention that became a common tool of hysteria doctors to produce "hysterical paroxysm" in women, there were impressive technological advances in the realm of prostate massage. In 1906, one doctor described his own self-designed, vibrating rectal electrostim device, complete with multiple vibration speeds! This may sound scary, but let's not forget that today there are many sex toys, including anal toys, that use a low level of electricity to add a touch of tingle. (See the "Electrostim" section in chapter 11, Toys.) The inventor of that device stated that the stimulation was not painful and when used correctly could be quite "soothing."[60]

Today, we know that the prostate is an erogenous zone for many men, and that massaging it can feel tremendously pleasurable and can lead to orgasm and ejaculation. In retrospect it is telling that prostate massage was once so prevalent as a medical treatment.

In *Tiresian Poetics: Modernism, Sexuality, Voice, 1888–2001*, Ed Madden compares the use of prostate massage and other forms of anal penetration in the medical context to the use of vibrators by doctors during the same time period: "If, as Rachel Maines demonstrates in *The Technology of Orgasm*, [...] doctors were producing orgasms in women to cure their nervous illness, then I think similar claims might be made for rectal dilators [and prostate massage]. Given [...] massage of the prostate to relieve neurasthenic 'congestion,' the use of dilation to cure nocturnal emissions, the use of electrodes in the anus for neurasthenia, and given the repeated emphasis on 'relief' that I find in the literature, I would argue that rectal dilators were also sexual devices employed for 'medical' reasons."[61] That is to say, in many cases, the medical procedure of prostate massage may have involved the doctor bringing the patient to ejaculation.

We are not suggesting that the doctors were getting off on it. The literature suggests that most doctors, and most patients, truly regarded the prostate massage as a medical procedure, in exactly the same way that massaging women with a vibrator on the clitoris to hysterical paroxysm (orgasm) was considered a medical procedure.

It's likely that many of the patients who sought out prostate massage believed they had a disease and may have suffered real anxiety over it. But there is evidence that at least some of them were wise to what was really happening during the medical procedure of "milking the prostate." One doctor said in 1917, "It often occurs that old men, no longer capable of performing the sexual act, will persist in coming to the physician for treatment, for the reason that they experience a sensation of sexual pleasure in having their prostate massaged. Especially is this true when the massage is continued to the point of forcing out the secretions (milking the prostate). Many of these old men secure all their sexual pleasures through these treatments."[62]

Another physician complained of patients who, after being cured of gonorrheal infection of the prostate, persist in wanting further treatment: "They return time and again to the clinics and state that while the pain or whatever it may be they complained of last time, has yielded to treatment; there is now something else. [...] one can never give them enough instrumental treatment. Many of them revel in being endo-scoped—they welcome the use of the Kollman [urethral] dilator—stripping of the vesicles, electrical and manual massage of the prostate and what not [...]."[63]

Certainly, in cases where doctors treated patients for chronic prostatitis, the massage was probably uncomfortable or even painful, given the compromised state of the gland. It is unlikely that men in this condition felt any pleasure during the massage.

But massage was also used to treat a number of "ailments" which, like hysteria, are no longer considered diseases, and which are also very sexual in nature. On the subject of hysteria, Maines suggested that the treatment was used to "cure" women of normal sexuality. Again, the same might be said for prostate massage: that it was used to treat normal male sexuality in an era of sexual repression. It was used to "cure" masturbation,[64] priapism,[65] and an overflow of blood to the prostate, which led to "erections on slight provocation, and an excessive growth of the sexual secretions which find their exit by frequent nocturnal pollutions" (aka wet dreams).[66]

Massage was also used for impotence,[67] premature ejaculation,[68] and "sexual neurasthenia" —a condition involving unstable emotions, various physical symptoms and, often, impotence.[69] Sexual neurasthenia shared a lot in common with hysteria, and similarly, most Western medical authorities no longer define it as a disease.

The Dawn of Antibiotics

The role of prostate massage in the medical industry changed when antibiotics came into the picture. By the late 1940s, antibiotics were frequently used for urethral infections,[70] which meant that most of these infections were cured before they could spread to the prostate, and by 1954 acute prostatitis (Type I) had "practically disappeared."[71] When an infection did spread from the urethra to the prostate and caused acute prostatitis, antibiotics proved very effective there as well. Antibiotics were already found to be "generally disappointing in treating chronic prostatitis," but even then, "an occasional case [...] responded dramatically."[72]

With such promising results, antibiotics quickly became the new first line of treatment for all kinds of prostatitis. Prostate massage fell out of favor and became increasingly infrequent as a medical practice. Some doctors continued to recommend it for particularly hard-to-cure cases of prostatitis as a last-ditch effort to ease symptoms, but most doctors stopped performing massage except as a means to collect prostatic fluid for testing.

Prostate Massage Makes a Comeback

To the frustration of many doctors and patients alike, even today most cases of CP/CPPS are not cured by antimicrobial medications. This has led to a resurgence of interest in prostate massage as a form of alternative or supplementary treatment for CP/CPPS. Some men who struggle with long-term cases of this condition have found that regularly repeated prostate massage affords them short-term symptom relief.

Anecdotal reports like these are listed at prostatitis.org, an online community of prostatitis patients, where many men describe giving themselves prostate massages at home or receiving them from their partners. They report total or partial relief of symptoms following massage when it is repeated 2–3 times per week.

Unfortunately, this does not cure the condition; it only eases the symptoms, which return if the massage is not continued on a regular basis. But this short-term relief can be a big improvement for those who struggle with annoying and painful come-and-go symptoms, sometimes for years. And in some cases, the combination of antibiotics and frequent, repeated prostate massage has brought about long-term symptom improvement. Dr. A.E. Feliciano Jr., a urologist with over 25 years of experience working with CP/CPPS and other genitourinary complaints at the Manila Clinic in the Philippines, has had much success in providing long-term relief to CP/CPPS patients through doctor-induced massage, culture-specific antibiotics, plus dietary and lifestyle changes.

In one study, Feliciano and others documented the treatment of 26 patients who had chronic, difficult-to-cure cases of prostatitis. The men were given prostate massages three times per week plus antibiotics or other medications for 6–12 weeks.[73] Their symptoms were rated with a series of questionnaires, and there was significant improvement in the average symptom severity. About 20 percent of the patients reported continued relief in follow-up two years later. This may seem like a small percentage, but for such hard-to-cure cases, to have even 20 percent gain lasting relief is a big deal.

Another group of medical professionals reported their results in treating 73 CP/CPPS patients with massage performed 1–3 times weekly, ranging from 2 to 12 weeks' duration, plus antibiotics. Follow-up ranged from 4 to 15 months, and a full 40 percent of these patients had complete symptom relief.[74]

These examples may seem promising, but the general consensus of the medical community is that further studies are necessary to determine the possible benefit of prostate massage for CP/CPPS. Even in the studies cited above, the combination of massage and antibiotics helps only for some patients, while others have little or no symptom improvement, so it's obviously not effective for everyone who gets lumped into this diagnosis.

As often happens, not all studies show the same results. In one, massage and antibiotics together were no more effective than antibiotics alone in treating CP/CPPS patients. In this study, patients were divided into two groups. For one month, the first group received massage three times weekly plus antibiotics, while the second group received antibiotics only. Because this study had a control group that did not receive the massage, it allows comparison of the results between those who received the massage and those who didn't in a way that isn't possible with retrospective studies. The results? There was improvement in both groups, but it was no greater in the massage group than in the no-massage group.[75]

Another factor may be the specific massage technique used. In one study patients were surveyed on how effective they thought prostate massage was in treating their prostate condition, and their responses indicated that they perceived a wide variation in the abilities of the physicians performing the massage.[76] This variation in technique may also come into play.

CAN MASSAGE HELP PREVENT PROSTATE CANCER?

Some experts speculate that prostate massage may help prevent prostate cancer. This theory is based on the idea that prostate massage can help clear the gland of irritants which may be involved in the development of cancer. Recent research indicates that inflammation, which occurs in many cases of prostatitis, may play an important and perhaps even causative role in the development of both BPH and prostate cancer: "Emerging evidence indicates that prostatic inflammation may contribute to prostate growth either in terms of hyperplastic (benign prostatic hyperplasia [BPH]) or neoplastic (prostate cancer) changes."[77]

The state of chronic inflammation alters the cellular environment within the glands of the prostate. Research under way suggests that lingering inflammatory products may play a role in the genome mutations that set the stage for cancer to develop, and perhaps BPH as well. Ironically, that means that the very presence of inflammation (which is a part of the body's defense mechanism) may in fact be causing harm.

If it is true that the state of chronic inflammation contributes to the development of BPH and prostate cancer, then prostate massage may help prevent

> *"It is today widely accepted that inflammation has a role in many human cancers."*
>
> —SONYA VASTO ET AL.

or delay the development of these diseases *if* it can reduce or prevent inflammation. Massage may help prevent inflammation from developing in the first place by "keeping the pipes clean." By flushing out the glands of the prostate, massage may help clear out irritants before they become a problem.

If inflammation is already happening, massage will help clear out the wastes of the inflammatory process (pus) by forcing them out manually and continually prompting the production of fresh prostatic fluid. This may not stop the inflammation, but at least it may keep inflammatory products from sitting there for prolonged periods. Also, massage supports circulation to the tissues and cells, and in this way encourages the natural healing process of the body.

And in cases where prostate massage can (in combination with antibiotics) cure prostatitis, it may be beneficial in reducing inflammation. However, it is not entirely clear that inflammation is always eliminated even in cases where symptoms subside.

In one study by Feliciano and colleagues, inflammation

was measured by counting white blood cells in the prostatic fluid while patients complaining of lower urinary tract symptoms were treated with regular massages and antimicrobials. Over the course of treatment, the white blood cell counts would increase to a peak, then drop again. The researchers suggested that this peak in white blood cell count is a sign that trapped pockets of infection were being opened, causing the release of the inflammatory product. If this is true, it may be very good for cancer prevention. However, there was no significant difference between the inflammation level at the start of treatment and at the end, even when symptoms were resolved.

So, it seems that even when massage plus antibiotics clears symptoms, it does not necessarily put an end to the inflammation, even though it may at least flush out trapped, inflamed pockets.

It is unclear whether prostate massage can reduce the risk of cancer or BPH. A causative relationship between inflammation and cancer/BPH has not yet been definitively proven, and even if it were, it is still unknown how prostate massage can affect your chances. More studies will be necessary before we can know what role prostate massage might play in prevention.

Regular prostate massage is not a replacement for prostate cancer screening. Even if it does help, it's no guarantee. Other factors come into play, such as age, genetic predisposition, race, and diet. But at the least, prostate massage potentially improves your odds, and you might just have a nice time while you're at it!

DIY PROSTATE MASSAGE FOR HEALTH

When prostate massage is performed for health reasons, typically the goal is to clear the gland of as much fluid as possible. This is sometimes called "draining" or "milking" the prostate. The technique is to position the finger on one side, apply pressure, and then slide toward the center, pushing the fluids from glands and ducts at the periphery toward the urethra at the midline. Repeat on the other side, once again starting on the outer edge and sliding toward the midline. You can cover the whole prostate this way, rubbing side-to-center on one side, then the other, and moving from top to bottom in this fashion.

If you want to massage your prostate to support the health of the gland, you can use your own fingers or a toy, or you can recruit someone else to do it for you. For guidelines on self-massage, see chapter 7, Find It: Locating the Gland. For toy tips, see chapter 11, Toys.

Sometimes the movement of fluid within the prostate can be felt by the finger. Drained fluids may appear at the tip of the penis, ranging from a single drop to an abundant flow. This may not happen every time you perform massage, and some men may never have any visible fluid. If the prostate feels tender, as it may for the first few times, go easy. You may be a little sore the next day. With repeated massages, this will happen less and less.

SOURCES OF QUOTES

Vibhash C. Mishra, John Browne, and Mark Emberton, "Role of Repeated Prostatic Massage in Chronic Prostatitis: A Systematic Review of the Literature," *Urology* 72.4 (2008), 732.

James Bayard Clark, *Essays on Genitourinary Subjects* (William Wood and Company, 1912), 121.

Sonya Vasto et al., "Inflammation and prostate cancer," *Future Oncology* 4.5 (2008): 637ff. (Academic OneFile, Aug. 13, 2010).

CONCLUSION

One of the most amazing things about sex is that there are so many ways to enjoy it. Unfortunately, sometimes people are so focused on one kind of sex that they forget about all the other options. While this can happen to anyone, it's especially common for men, for whom the focus on performance over pleasure often gets in the way.

No matter how many men and their partners we've talked with, it's always amazing to hear their excitement when they discover how good it feels to play with the prostate. And as more guys try it out and see that it can be a great addition to an exciting sex life, there's more discussion of it in the world.

We hope that as the erogenous nature of the prostate gets more attention, more research will study the role of the prostate in male erotic pleasure. We are also very eager to see what research may show about the possible benefits of massage to prostate health. But even if prostate massage doesn't turn out to prevent cancer, we know that there are lots of other reasons to do it!

No matter where you are in your explorations of P-spot play, whether you're starting out or you've been enjoying it for years, there's always something new to discover. We hope that this book has been a useful guide for you and that you've found new ways to experience pleasure. And remember—it doesn't mean you can't also have fun in the ways you're used to. We're just adding a few more options to the menu.

With pleasure,
Charlie Glickman and Aislinn Emirzian

AFTERWORD

Although many generations of women and men have attempted to understand and describe their sexual experiences through art, literature, and observation, the systematic study of human sexuality is quite young. Pioneering researcher Dr. Alfred Kinsey and his colleagues at Indiana University—where I've been privileged to work for over a decade—first began their interview-based studies of sexual behavior in the 1930s.

The "youth" of this science—combined with social constructions of masculinity and historical taboos related to homosexuality and sexual behavior—mean that certain sexual behaviors, such as prostate stimulation and pleasuring, are largely understudied. We know a great deal—though certainly not everything—about penile-vaginal intercourse and oral sex, including how many American women and men engage in these behaviors; the extent to which vaginal and oral sex generally feel pleasurable or arousing; how often they're connected to orgasm for women and men; the ages at which people commonly first begin having vaginal inter-course or oral sex; and how people incorporate sex toys into these types of sexual expression.

Yet, from a scientific perspective, we don't know any of this about prostate stimulation. Research related to prostate stim-ulation is very rarely conducted and is mostly limited to select groups of men (such as men who have sex with men), which leaves many curious men and their partners in the dark. This is especially true for men who only or mostly have sex with women and who may not have a group of male friends among whom they feel comfortable talking about prostate play.

Let's say, for example, that you're a straight-identified man who has heard that prostate play feels good. Where do you go to learn more about it? What are the chances that you have a friend, brother, or dad whom you can ask about stimulating your own prostate, choosing anal toys for masturbation or use with a partner, or how to even find and stimulate your prostate in the first place?

Most straight-identified men I know and have heard from for years in my work as a sex columnist and sexuality educator feel like they don't have many—if any—friends they can ask these kinds of questions. For many men, their only experi-ences talking about their prostate or having it touched are in the context of clinical exams as they get older. This is a shame, considering the potential for pleasure that lies within.

And yet it's possible that one or more of their best guy friends—or yes, even one of their family members—regularly engages in prostate play. They're likely just not as vocal about it as men often are about masturbation, vaginal sex, or receiving oral sex.

All this means that prostate pleasuring may or may not be rarely practiced (given the lack of research on the topic, we don't know how rare or common it is among men in the United States)—but it's certainly a largely invisible practice. Fortunately, the recent mainstreaming of sex toys, including some prostate-specific toys, has made some men and women more aware of prostate play. In the past decade, we've also seen more discussion about prostate play by men of all sexual orientations (as well as some transgender women who have prostates) in mainstream sex columns, including columns by me, Dan Savage, and others who write about sex.

Authors and sexuality educators Charlie Glickman and Aislinn Emirzian have assembled a wealth of knowledge, suggestions, and advice from people they've talked with over the years that should be helpful to many men and women who are curious about prostate stimulation—as well as to those who are seasoned in the practice and looking for new perspectives, techniques, or ideas for their private or partnered play.

I work as a sexuality researcher and educator because, although I know a great deal about sex, I don't know everything about it (no one does)—and I enjoy learning from others. In reading *The Ultimate Guide to Prostate Pleasure*, I appreciate that I was exposed to new ways of thinking about prostate stimulation and to perspectives that Charlie and Aislinn have gleaned from others' trials, errors, and significant pleasures. This very good book will likely influence many people's sexual lives, and ways of thinking about sex and what it means to be a man (and a sexual man) for years to come.

Debby Herbenick, PhD, MPH
Bloomington, Indiana

RESOURCES

PROSTATE PLAY GUIDES

Tantric Male Multiple G-spot Orgasm, by Somraj Pokras and Jeffre TallTrees (Tantra at Tahoe, 2003)

The Healthy Prostate
www.thehealthyprostate.com
Lots of great info and instructional videos available for download

Pleasure Mechanics
www.pleasuremechanics.com
Excellent how-to videos, including *Pleasure Mechanics Guide to Prostate Massage: How to Enjoy Pleasurable & Healthy Prostate Stimulation*

MALE MULTIPLE ORGASM

The Multi-Orgasmic Man: Sexual Secrets Every Man Should Know, by Mantak Chia and Douglas Abrams (HarperOne, 1997)

The Multi-Orgasmic Couple: Sexual Secrets Every Couple Should Know, by Mantak Chia et al. (HarperOne, 2001)

Any Man Can, by William Hartman and Marilyn Fithian (St. Martins Mass Market Paper, 1986)

Orgasm: New Dimensions, by Prakash Kothari (VRP Publishers, 1989)

ESO: How You and Your Lover Can Give Each Other Hours of Extended Sexual Orgasm, by Alan P. Brauer and Donna J. Brauer (Grand Central Publishing, 2001)

The Body Electric School www.thebodyelectricschool.com

Experiential workshops on Tantra, massage, and erotic practices

ANAL PLAY

Anal Pleasure and Health, 4th ed., by Jack Morin (Down There Press, 2010)

The Ultimate Guide to Anal Sex for Men, by Bill Brent (Cleis Press, 2002)

The Ultimate Guide to Anal Sex for Women, 2nd ed., by Tristan Taormino (Cleis Press, 2006)

Anal Massage for Lovers Vol. 2, directed by Joseph Kramer (Joseph Kramer Productions, 2006, 160 minutes)

Anal Massage for Relaxation and Pleasure, directed by Joseph Kramer (Pacific Media, 2007, 160 minutes)

Bend Over Boyfriend, directed by Shar Rednour (Fatale Video, 1998, 60 minutes)

Bend Over Boyfriend 2: More Rockin' Less Talkin', directed by Shar Rednour and Jackie Strano (S.I.R. Video, 1999, 70 minutes)

Expert Guide to Anal Pleasure for Men, directed by Tristan Taormino (Vivid-Ed, 2010, 102 minutes)

The Expert Guide to Pegging, directed by Tristan Taormino (Vivid-Ed, 2012, 129 minutes)

Tickle My Tush, by Sadie Allison (Tickle Kitty Press, 2011)

Uranus: Self Anal Massage for Men, directed by Joseph Kramer (Joseph Kramer Productions, 2004, 100 minutes)

FISTING

Trust: The Hand Book: A Guide to the Sensual and Spiritual Art of Handballing, by Bert Herrman (Alamo Square Press, 1991)

G-SPOT PLAY

Expert Guide to the G-Spot, directed by Tristan Taormino (Vivid-Ed, 2007, 80 minutes)

Female Ejaculation and the G-Spot, by Debbie Sundahl (Hunter House, 2003)

The G-Spot and Other Discoveries about Human Sexuality, by Alice Kahn Ladas, Beverly Whipple, and John D. Perry (Holt Paperbacks, 2004)

GUSH: The Official Guide to the G-Spot & Female Ejaculation (Good Releasing, 2011, 90 minutes)

ELECTRICITY PLAY

Juice: Electricity for Pleasure and Pain, by Uncle Abdul
   (Greenery Press, 1998)

FINDING A DOCTOR

Gay and Lesbian Medical Association
http://www.glma.org/index.cfm?fuseaction=Page.viewPage
   &pageId=939&grandparentID=534&parentID=938&no
   deID=1
A database of primary care providers, specialists, therapists,
   dentists, and other health professionals who are welcoming
   to LGBTQ patients
Kink-Aware Professionals
https://ncsfreedom.org/resources/kink-aware-professionals-
   directory/kap-directory-homepage.html
A database of doctors, therapists, and lawyers who are sensitive to diverse forms of sexuality

PROSTATE HEALTH

*Dr. Katz's Guide to Prostate Health: From Conventional to
   Holistic Therapies*, by Aaron Katz (Freedom Press, 2006)
*The Prostate Health Program: A Guide to Preventing and
   Controlling Prostate Cancer*, by Daniel W. Nixon and
   Max Gomez (Free Press, 2004)
A Gay Man's Guide to Prostate Cancer, by Gerald Perlman
   and Jack Drescher (Informa Healthcare, 2005)
*A Headache in the Pelvis: A New Understanding and Treat-
   ment for Prostatitis and Chronic Pelvic Pain Syndromes*,

6th ed., by David Wise and Rodney Anderson (National Center for Pelvic Pain Research, 2012)

Male Care

www.malecare.org

A resource and support group for men with cancer—organizes support groups for gay men

American Cancer Society

www.cancer.org

The book *Sexuality for the Man with Cancer* is available free on the society's website and has lots of great info about prostate cancer and sex.

The Prostate Cancer Foundation

www.prostatecancerfoundation.org

The Prostate Cancer Infolink

www.prostatecancerinfolink.net/

The Prostatitis Foundation

www.prostatitis.org

PLACES TO BUY TOYS

Adam & Eve

www.adamandeve.com, 800-293-4654

Mail order and online store

Aneros

www.aneros.com

Creators of the Aneros, the unique prostate massage toy

Babeland

www.babeland.com, 800-658-9119

Sex-positive retail and online store, with locations in Seattle
and New York

Come As You Are

www.comeasyouare.com, 877-858-3160

Sex-positive retail and online sex toy company with a store in
Toronto

Good Vibrations

www.goodvibes.com, 800-289-8423

Sex-positive retail and online store, with locations in San
Francisco, Oakland, Berkeley, and Boston

JT Stockroom

www.stockroom.com, 800-755-8697

Sex-positive retail and online company, with a store in Los
Angeles. A great source of BDSM gear.

Liberator Shapes

www.liberator.com

Makers of excellent supports designed to make sexual positions easier

Lube Shooter

www.lubeshooter.com

Lube shooters make it easier to get lube where you want it.

Mr. S Leather

www.mr-s-leather.com, 800-746-7677

Retail and online store specializing in BDSM gear with a store in San Francisco

She Bop

www.sheboptheshop.com, 503-473-8018

Sex-positive retail and online company with a store in Portland, Oregon

Smitten Kitten

www.smittenkittenonline.com, 888-751-0523

Sex-positive retail and online company with a store in Minneapolis

Venus Envy

www.venusenvy.ca, 877-370-9288

Sex-positive retail and online company with stores in Ottawa and Halifax

GENERAL INFORMATION

San Francisco Sex Information

www.sfsi.org, 415-989-7374

Free, anonymous, nonjudgmental information and referrals

www.sexuality.about.com

Excellent information on a wide range of sexuality topics
written by Cory Silverberg, an amazing sex educator

The American Association of Sexuality Educators, Counselors, and Therapists www.aasect.org

If you're looking for a sex therapist, AASECT is a great place
to look for referrals and information.

ENDNOTES

Chapter 3

1 Peter T. Scardino and Judith Kelman, *Dr. Peter Scardino's Prostate Book: The Complete Guide to Overcoming Prostate Cancer, Prostatitis, and BPH* (Penguin, 2006), 12.

2 Ibid.

3 The "Sacred Gate" refers to the female G-spot in Tantric circles.

4 "Ejaculatory Physiology and Dysfunction," *Urology clinics of North America,* vol. 2, 363–75, 2001.

5 Alice Kahn Ladas, Beverly Whipple, and John D. Perry, *The G Spot and Other Recent Discoveries about Human Sexuality* (Dell Publishing, 1982), 33.

6   Ibid., 28.

7   Amichai Kilchevsky, Yoram Vardi, Lior Lowenstein, and Ilan Gruenwald, "Is the Female G-Spot Truly a Distinct Anatomic Entity?" *Journal of Sexual Medicine*, vol. 9, issue 3 (March 2012), 719–726.

8   Ibid., 721–722; Terence M. Hines, "The G-spot: A modern gynecologic myth," *American Journal of Obstetrics and Gynecology*, vol. 185 (2001), 359–362.

9   Pierre Foldes and Odile Buisson, "The Clitoral Complex: A Dynamic Sonographic Study," *Journal of Sexual Medicine*, vol. 6, issue 5 (May 2009), 1223–1231.

10 Ladas et al., 53.

11 Ibid., 137.

Chapter 5

12 R. Louis Schultz, *Out in the Open: the Complete Male Pelvis* (North Atlantic Books, 1999), 11.

13 Jack Morin, *Anal Pleasure and Health*, 3rd ed. (Down There Press, 1998), 67.

Chapter 7

14 Lisa Marr, *Sexually Transmitted Diseases: A Physician Tells You What You Need to Know*, 2nd ed. (Johns Hopkins University Press, 2007), 32.

15 Ibid., 32–33.

Chapter 9

16 Somraj Pokras and Jeffre TallTrees, *Tantric Male Multiple G-Spot Orgasm* (Tantra at Tahoe, 2003), 120.

Chapter 11

17 www.aneros.com.

Chapter 12

18 Morin, *Anal Pleasure and Health*, 104.

19 Karlyn Lotney, *The Ultimate Guide to Strap-On Sex: A Complete Resource for Women and Men* (Cleis Press, 2000), 68.

Chapter 13

20 *Cisgender* refers to people who experience and present their gender in a way that is aligned with the gender they were assigned at birth. It is contrasted with *transgender*, which refers to people who experience their gender as different from the gender they were assigned, and who may take a variety of steps to bring them into alignment.

21 The word *punk* has a few different meanings. It can mean a person with a mohawk, as in "punk rock." It can mean a loser. And it can mean a gay man, especially if he's effeminate or on the receiving end of penetration. This last definition is more common in African American communities.

22 *Maricón* is a Spanish term that refers to the man on the receiving end of anal sex from another man. It has connotations of effeminacy and is often used as an insult or a slur.

Chapter 14

23 Steven Morganstern and Allen Abrahams, *The Prostate Sourcebook*, 3rd ed. (Lowellhouse, 1998), xi.

24 Thomas A. Stamey, *Pathogenesis and Treatment of Urinary Tract Infections* (Williams and Wilkins, 1980), 343.

25 Aaron E. Katz, *Dr. Katz's Guide to Prostate Health: From Conventional to Holistic Therapies* (Freedom Press, 2006), 57.

26 http://www.ncbi.nlm.nih.gov/pmc/articles/PMC1476089/.

27 Sonya Vasto et al., "Inflammation and prostate cancer," *Future Oncology* 4.5 (2008): 637ff. (Academic OneFile, Aug. 13, 2010).

28 Alessandro Sciarra, Franco Di Silverio, Stefano Salciccia, Ana Maria Autran Gomez, Alessandro Gentilucci, and Vincenzo Gentile, "Inflammation and Chronic Prostatic Diseases: Evidence for a Link?" *European Urology* 52.4 (2007): 964ff. (Academic OneFile, Aug. 13, 2010).

29 www.thehealthyprostate.com.

30 Daniel W. Nixon and Max Gomez, *The Prostate Health Program: A Guide to Preventing and Controlling Prostate Cancer* (Free Press, 2004), 174.

31 M. Gover, "A Statistical study of the etiology of benign hypertrophy of the prostate gland," *Johns Hopkins Hospital Reports* 1923;21:231–295.

32 Katz, *Dr. Katz's Guide to Prostate Health*, 13.

33 Nixon and Gomez, *The Prostate Health Program*, 170.

34 Ernani Luis Rhoden and Abraham Morgantaler, "Risks of Testosterone-Replacement Therapy and Recommendations for Monitoring," *New England Journal of Medicine* 350 (2004), 482–492.

35 http://www.cancer.org/Cancer/ProstateCancer/ DetailedGuide/prostate-cancer-risk-factors.

36 http://www.cancer.org/Cancer/ProstateCancer/ DetailedGuide/prostate-cancer-detection.

37 Marie-Blanche Tchetgen, James T. Song, Myla Strawderman, Steven J. Jacobsen and Joseph E. Oesterling, "Ejaculation Increases the Serum Prostate-specific Antigen Concentration," *Urology*, vol. 47, issue 4 (1996), 511–516.

38 Thomas A. Stamey, Norman Yang, Alan R. Hay, John E. McNeal, Fuad S. Freiha, and Elise Redwine, "Prostate-Specific Antigen as a Serum Marker for Adenocarcinoma of the Prostate," *New England Journal of Medicine* 317 (1987), 909–916.

39 Francesco Montorsi, Gerald Brock, Jay Lee, JoAnn Shapiro, Hendrik Van Poppel, Markus Graefen, and Christian Stief, "Effect of Nightly versus On-Demand Vardenafil on Recovery of Erectile Function in Men Following Bilateral Nerve-Sparing Radical Prostatectomy," *European Urology* 54 (2008), 924–931.

40 Nixon and Gomez, *The Prostate Health Program*, 169.

41 Ibid., 170.

42 Stephen E. Goldstone, "The Ups and Downs of Gay Sex After Prostate Cancer Treatment," in *A Gay Man's Guide to Prostate Cancer*, Gerald Perlman and Jack Drescher, eds. (Haworth Medical Press, 2005), 47.

43 M. Koeman, M.F. van Driel, W.C.M. Weijmar Schultz, and H.J.A. Mensink, "Orgasm after radical prostatectomy," *British Journal of Urology*, vol. 77 (1996), 861–864.

44 Ibid.

Chapter 15

45 Thomas S. Keener, Thomas C. Winter, Richard Berger, John N. Krieger, Cynthia Nodell, Ivan Rothman, and Hanh V. Nghiem, "Prostate Vascular Flow: The Effect of Ejaculation as Revealed on Transrectal Power Doppler Sonography," *American Journal of Roentgenology* 2000;175:1169-1172 (abstract), http://www.ajronline.org/cgi/content/full/175/4/1169.

46 David Wise and Rodney Anderson, *A Headache in the Pelvis: A New Understanding and Treatment for Prostatitis and Chronic Pelvic Pain Syndromes*, 4th ed. (National Center for Pelvic Pain Research, 2006), 91.

47 R.U. Anderson, D. Wise, T. Sawyer, P. Glowe, E.K. Orenberg, "6-day intensive treatment protocol for refractory chronic prostatitis/chronic pelvic pain syndrome using myofascial release and paradoxical relaxation training," *Journal of Urology*, April 2011;185(4):1294–9 (Epub Feb 22, 2011), http://www.ncbi.nlm.nih.gov/pubmed/21334027.

48 Nixon and Gomez, *The Prostate Health Program*, 171.

49 http://www.prostatitis.org/a162000.html.

50 G.F. Lydston, "Massage of the Prostate," *Physician and Surgeon*, vol. 17 (J.W. Keating, 1895), 281.

51 Ibid., 282.

52 Bernard Simon Talmey, *Neurasthenia Sexualis: a Treatise on Sexual Impotence in Men and in Women* (Practitioners' Pub. Co., 1912), 147.

53 William Josephus Robinson, *A Practical Treatise on the Causes, Symptoms, and Treatment of Sexual Impotence*

and other Sexual Disorders in Men and Women (Critic and Guide, 1913), 213–214.

54 Ibid., 345.

55 Ibid., 213–214.

56 George Frank Lydston, *Impotence and Sterility: With Aberrations of the Sexual Function and Sex-Gland Implantation* (Riverton Press, 1917), 203.

57 http://wiki.malegspot.com/index.php?title=Aneros_ History; http://www.chron.com/disp/story.mpl/metropolitan/7036873.html.

58 Ed Madden, *Tiresian Poetics: Modernism, Sexuality, Voice, 1888–2001* (Associated University Presses, 2008), 159.

59 Lydston, "Massage of the Prostate," 281.

60 George Whitfield Overall, *A Non-surgical Treatise on Diseases of the Prostate Gland and Adnexa*, 2nd ed. (Rowe Pub. Co., 1906), 102b.

61 Madden, *Tiresian Poetics*, 159.

62 Franklyn Pierre Davis, *Impotency, Sterility, and Artificial Impregnation* (Mosby, 1917), 74.

63 Frederic S. Mason, "Post-Gonorrhoeal Neurasthenia," *Urologic and Cutaneous Review*, vol. 21 (Urologic & Cutaneous Press, 1917), 319.

64 Iwan Bloch, *The Sexual Life of Our Time in Its Relations to Modern Civilization* (Forgotten Books), translated from German.

65 Robinson, *A Practical Treatise on the Causes, Symptoms, and Treatment of Sexual Impotence*, 345.

66 L. Bolton Bangs, "On the Treatment of Some Genito-Urinary Maladies," *Medical Brief*, vol. 32, issue 2 (1904), 551.

67 Talmey, *Neurasthenia Sexualis*, 147.

68 Robinson, *A Practical Treatise on the Causes, Symptoms, and Treatment of Sexual Impotence*, 213–214.

69 Mason, "Post-Gonorrhoeal Neurasthenia," 319.

70 Frank Henry Netter, *The Ciba Collection of Medical Illustrations: A Compilation of Pathological and Anatomical Paintings*, vol. 2 (Ciba Pharmaceutical Products, 1948).

71 Meredith Fairfax Campbell, *Urology: Volume 1* (W.B. Saunders Co., 1954), 635.

72 Fletcher H. Colby, *Essential Urology* (Williams & Wilkins, 1956), 427.

73 J.C. Nickel, J. Downey, A.E. Feliciano Jr., and B. Hennenfent, "Repetitive Prostatic Massage Therapy for Chronic Refractory Prostatitis: The Philippine Experience," *Tech Urol.* 1999;5:146–151 (abstract), http://www.prostatitis.org/99workshop/Abstracts/abstract10/abstract10.html.

74 D.A. Shoskes and S.I. Zeitlin, "Use of prostatic massage in combination with antibiotics in the treatment of chronic prostatitis," *Prostate Cancer and Prostatic Diseases* 1999;2, 159–162.

75 Ahmad Ateya, Ashraf Fayez, Ragab Hani, Wael Zohdy, Mohammad A. Gabbar, and Rany Shamloul, "Evaluation of Prostatic Massage in Treatment of Chronic Prostatitis," *Urology* 2006;67:674–678.

76 B.R. Hennenfent and C.J. Hickman, "Patient-perceived Efficacy of Prostatic Massage as a Treatment Modality for Prostatitis, Prostatodynia, and BPH: An Exploratory Study," *Infections in Urology* 2000;13(6):148–164 (abstract), http://www.prostatitis.org/99workshop/

Abstracts/abstract13/abstract13.html.

77 Sciarra et al., "Inflammation and Chronic Prostatic Diseases," 964.

ABOUT THE AUTHORS

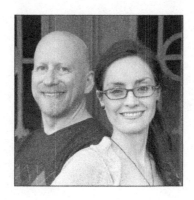

CHARLIE GLICKMAN is a sexuality educator, writer, blogger, and teacher. He has presented workshops on topics such as sex positivity, sex and shame, gender and masculinity, communities of erotic affiliation, and a wide range of sexual and relationship practices including prostate play, cock and ball play, polyamory, BDSM, sex toys, and safer sex. Charlie has also taught university courses for therapists and seminary students to help them provide the best sexual counseling for their clients, and he has presented at many conferences and community events. He is certified by the American Association of Sexuality Educators, Counselors, and Therapists (www.aasect.org) and is the Education Program Manager at Good Vibrations (www.goodvibes.

com). You can find out more about him and read his blog at www.charlieglickman.com.

While attending Smith College, **AISLINN EMIRZIAN** served as a peer sexuality educator for two years, teaching workshops to fellow students. Following graduation, she got involved with Oh My Sensuality Shop in Massachusetts and, later, Good Vibrations in California. During her years as a sex educator, she has taught workshops on a wide range of topics relating to sexuality, but the prostate is her favorite.

Photograph by Michael McAreavy.

INDEX